Vol. II

MW00959007

~ Written and Produced by:
Jamie Whyte MD
Dominic Mineo

~ Clinically approved and recommended by:

University/Salk Institute Scientist
Jamie Whyte MD

~ Dhurva® Models:

Stephania Ochs
Sofie Blicher
Laryn Finnegan
Shelby Lawson
Rachel Mulvaney
Crystal Richter
Dean Cortez
Jennifer Butler
Zsofia Illes
Yoshi Mayeaux
Dominic Mineo

~ Photo Locations:

Fit Athletic Club
M2i

Social media :
FB – Best Yoga Prop
IG - @bestyogaprop
DhurvaYoga.com

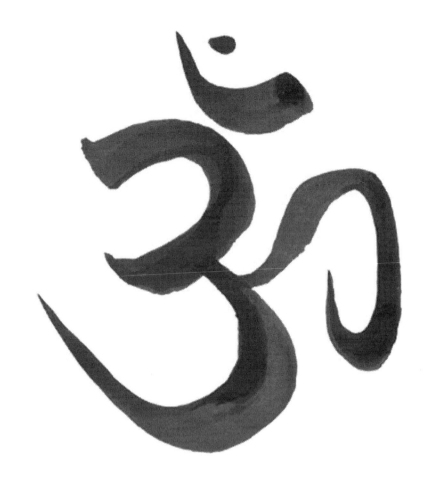

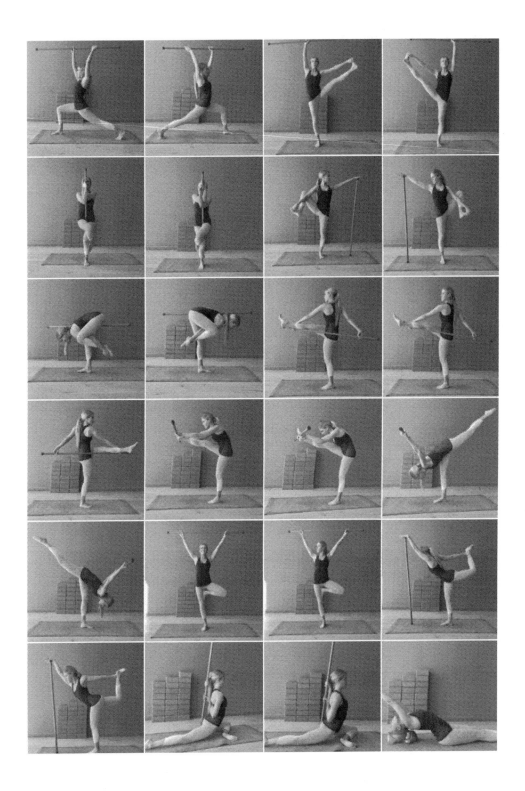

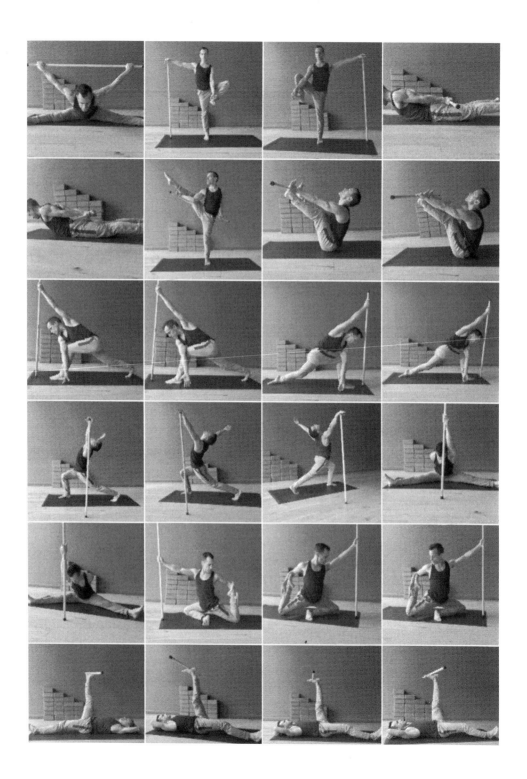

Jamie Whyte – *Author and Physician*

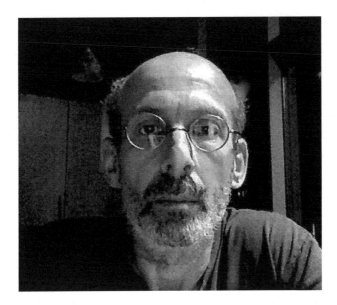

-BIOGRAPHY-

Dr. Whyte began his professional life in industry, working for his family's manufacturing concern. After the business was sold he took up the study of medicine, ultimately earning his M.D. and becoming a Director of the Sleep Disorders Center at Columbia-Presbyterian Medical Center in New York City. After several years of professional practice, he pursued an interest in law, obtaining a J.D. degree via the Law, Science and Technology program at Arizona State University. Then it was a move further west and back to science after being awarded a microbiology fellowship at the Salk Institute in La Jolla, California. There, Dr. Whyte conducted research on the interactions among exercise, metabolism and aging. Now on his fourth career, Dr. Whyte is currently a writer and entrepreneur based in San Diego

-YOGA AND FITNESS PHILOSOPHY-

In fitness, as elsewhere, balance and harmony are the essentials. And in this regard yoga is unique among all forms of physical activity. The yogic philosophy acknowledges excellence, but this recognition is aspirational, not competitive. It is uninhibited in its appreciation of the human form while avoiding the destructive obsession with physical appearance. A thoughtful practice almost magically integrates and harmonizes physicalism with spiritualism. Modern yoga expresses the wisdom of millennia yet still remains an openness to new forms and new ideas. If not a perfect system of exercise, yoga is the closest thing that we mortals have thus far devised.

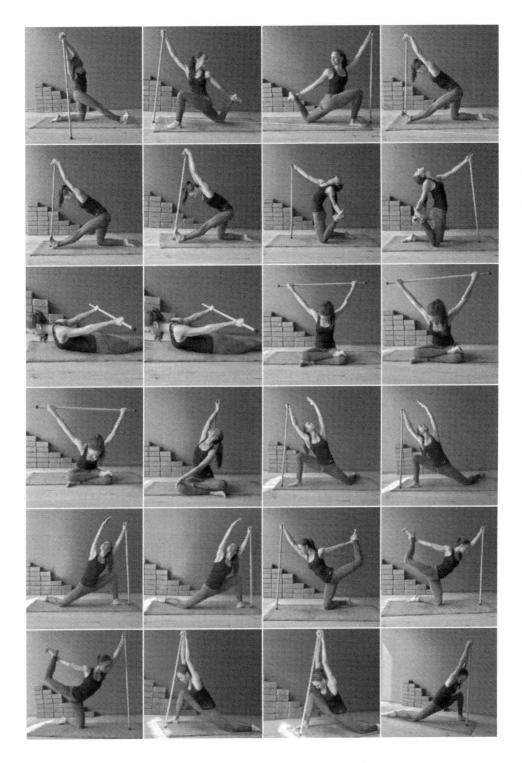

Dominic Mineo – *Author and Founder*

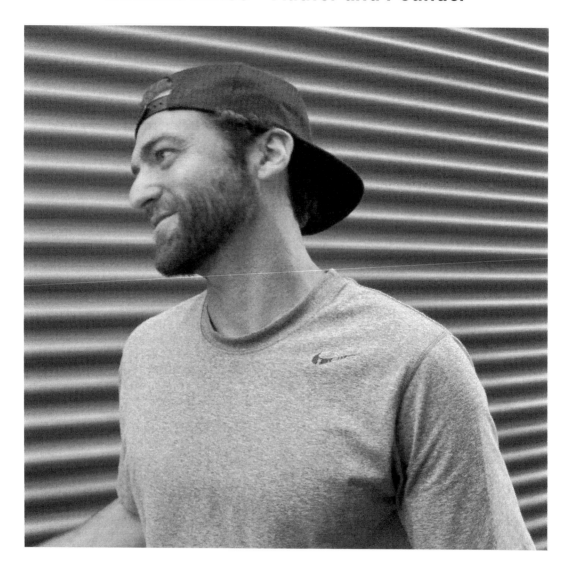

-BIOGRAPHY-

My interest in natural healing and caring for my body brought me to Yoga.
Fascinated by the unique physical challenge and sudden mental clarity from self
awareness, I enrolled in a teacher training program.
I spent the next the next 8 years teaching and practicing in over 50 countries and
all seven continents. Time forward, I'm now broadcasting the Dhurva Yoga® brand
across the globe making body therapy a necessity for self-care.

-YOGA AND FITNESS PHILOSOPHY-

I personally practice and teach functional movement Yoga. These movements
induce a strong, flexible base through gymnastic core strength using articulate
hand and foot balance.
Meditation, calmness and practicing patience promote a healing relaxed state which
enables focus and attention span to grow. Meditation also makes you aware, that
your inner attitude determines your happiness.
Committing to these understandings, one will embody a boost in immunity,
balanced metabolism, better sleep, a boost in sexual performance, weight
reduction, increased energy and vitality.
I am humbled and forever grateful for the opportunities given, and currently
offered, to teach the timelessness gift of Yoga.

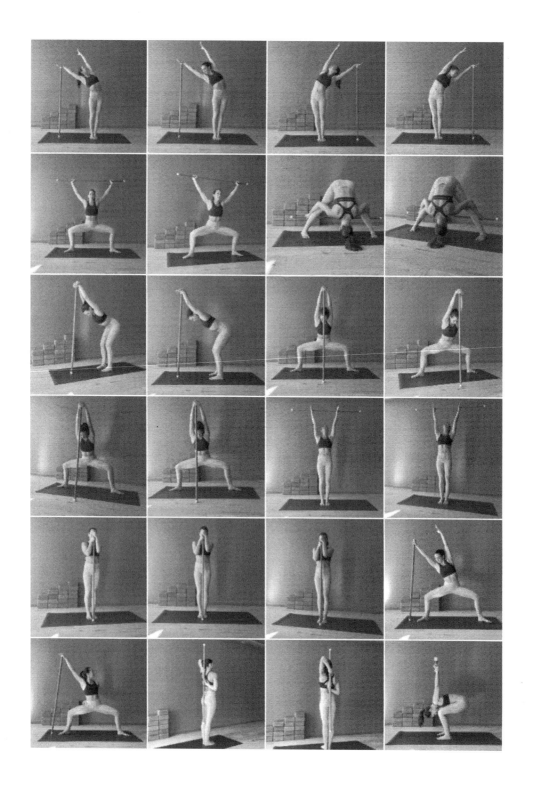

X

Table of Contents

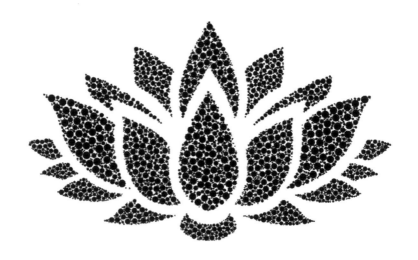

CHAPTER 1
FROM YOGA TO DHURVA

YOGA

When we speak of yoga we need to be mindful of our meaning. Indeed, the world of yoga is remarkably diverse. There are numerous forms ranging from the tranquil path of Hatha; to the spirited road of Ashtanga; to the scorching trail of Bikram. But these established forms are only the beginning. Change is ever present and yoga practice now includes a growing diversity of styles. Some of these novel incarnations are slight variations upon traditional themes. In some newer versions, however, even the most venerable tenets of practice are put to test. Novel, yoga-inspired activities such as competitive posing have even raised fundamental questions about what yoga is — or should be.

But despite all the novelty and diversity, several threads of the classical tapestry almost always remain. Purists have gone so far as to suggest that some of the newer forms be excluded from the yoga community. On this point, however, I tend to be less dogmatic. As long as the essentials are present, the practice has a place in the family of yogic forms. These essential elements still bind all of the yogic arts together and define the basis for an inclusive yoga community. I will describe these elements and discuss them in historical perspective, then briefly explain how Dhurva relates to both the centuries old traditions as well as the modern embellishments.

Breathing

Breathing, of course, is essential to human life. In our day-to-day lives we tend, though, to give breathing little conscious attention. It is performed automatically, even as we sleep. So unless disease or accident disrupts the natural rhythm, we generally pay little mind.

Historically, Western medicine has taken an unrefined view towards breathing. Yes, respiratory rate and depth are used as clinical indicators. Nevertheless, to a first approximation it acknowledges only a simple dichotomy, to wit, that you are either breathing or you aren't. In the first case all is well and in the second there is a dire emergency. The physiology of breathing, though, is far more nuanced and complex. Only recently have we in the West come around (better late than never!) to appreciate, at least in part, the importance of breathing properly in health as well as disease states.

Yogis, conversely, have long recognized that breathing, particularly under conditions of stress, is amenable to useful control by the application of technique. Thus, learning how to breathe properly is a mainstay of yoga instruction. In fact, this focus differentiates yoga from many other forms of athletic training. Centuries of experience have informed such instruction so that yoga is preeminent in using the breath as a means to enhance human health and overall well-being.

Acknowledging the centrality of breath control in virtually all forms of yoga, it should be recognized that different schools of yoga have their own approach to the subject. Traditionally, highly refined techniques (including, for example, single nostril breathing) are an element of the eightfold path to enlightenment originally articulated by the famed Yogi Patanjali. Many yogic forms, however, take a more down to earth approach and Dhurva is among them. Our emphasis is upon proper breathing techniques during posing and other physical activity as well as breathing as a focal point during meditation. That this approach is less ethereal than that of Patanjali, however, does not make it any less central to practice.

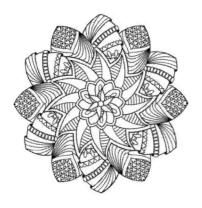

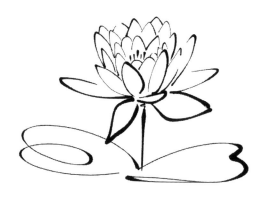

Stretching

Just as Western traditions have tended to view breathing as something of limited interest in the absence of overt disease, stretching too has been considered a technique with limited value. To be sure, stretching has importance to athletes who require great flexibility, e.g., gymnasts, ice hockey goalies and martial artists. But for non-athletes the virtues of stretching have been generally overlooked.

The traditional Western approach has been to use stretching as a warm-up in advance of exercise. The theory is that muscles and tendons need to be stretched in advance of activity to prevent injury. Indeed, this idea makes intuitive sense. Soft tissue pre-conditioned to states of stretch should, it would seem, be better able to withstand the rigors of actual competition.

Human physiology, however, often operates in counterintuitive fashion. Actual study of warm-up stretching has shown that the practice prior to athletic activity does not make injury less likely. If anything — and quite surprisingly — stretching for this purpose may be as likely to cause injury as actual competition. And the use of forceful, so-called ballistic stretches has especially been identified as a cause of injury in athletes, rather than being a useful preventative measure.

The Eastern approach towards stretching is very different. According to this traditional paradigm, stretching is a valuable exercise in itself, not simply a form of warm-up. Thus, one would never do demanding stretching poses at the start of a yoga class and then progress to poses which required strength and endurance. Rather, the yogi will instruct his students to begin by warming the body and only then proceed with poses which include challenges to range of motion.

In parallel with its unique emphasis upon the breath, yoga has a long tradition of focus upon stretching. Maintaining range of motion, flexibility in the hips and shoulders, as well as limberness in other joints has been a primary goal of a yoga practice. Perhaps most important, stretching is seen as an activity not suited only to competitive athletes. Instead, the flexibility gained from yoga is seen to have great benefit to everyone, serious athlete or not. It is this broad view of the utility of stretching which is characteristic of virtually all forms of yoga. Dhurva embraces this wisdom.

Meditation

Traditionally, Western science has been skeptical about meditation. But once again yoga was ahead of the curve. The health benefits of meditation are now being confirmed by modern science. Dozens of carefully performed studies show the profound influence that meditation can have upon human physiology. Only the most hidebound continue to believe that meditation has no place in our daily lives.

Dhurva uses meditation in for two very different — in fact, nearly opposite — purposes. First, we employ meditation to clear the mind completely of all thoughts. It is thus a means to help reset one's mental registers; to filter out those influences which cloud one's thinking and inhibit mental calm and clarity.
In this application meditation briefly removes consciousness from the cares and concerns that comprise daily life outside the yoga classroom. Strong feelings are muted and biases are released.

Second, meditation can provide a space for unimpeded thought. The process also includes the function to cool the flames of strong emotion and exclude extraneous thought. But rather than emptying the mind of all content, this form of meditation allows a laser-like focus upon a particular issue of concern. During this active meditation, one can introspect without interference from distorting, outside influences. Such meditation is a means to access one's true feelings and bring them to bear upon real world problems. The meditative state is thus a tool for introspection, analysis and problem-solving; for clarifying one's thoughts and feelings.

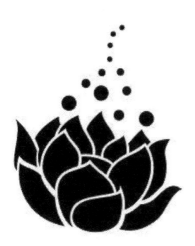

Strength and Endurance

Non-practitioners often have a stereotyped view of yoga, conjuring images of students sitting in lotus position intoning mantras; or perhaps twisted like a pretzel into some physics-defying contortion. But as real-life yogis know, these stereotypes — even to the extent that they contain a grain of truth — fail to recognize a central aim of yoga practice: improvement in strength and endurance.

So while it is true that yoga does not produce students who have the appearance or brute strength of a powerlifter, experienced yogis are remarkably strong and will often outperform competitive athletes when strength and endurance are measured. This comes as a surprise to the uninitiated, who know only the stereotypes and can't imagine the physical prowess to which yoga can lead.

This pinched view of yoga, though, is gradually disappearing. Sophisticated coaches and trainers have come to fully appreciate this aspect of yoga, incorporating poses and sometimes even a full yoga practice into the training regimes of elite athletes. Yoga is now used by triathletes, runners, swimmers, skiers and others — and not just for its more traditional use as an aid to flexibility and balance. By carefully selecting and sequencing yoga poses, both strength and endurance can be directly enhanced.

Importantly, one need not be an elite athlete to appreciate and benefit from yoga's capacity to improve these parameters. Practitioners at all fitness levels can receive this benefit. Yoga can even be used by physical therapists to improve strength and endurance in those with physical challenges as, for example, in the rehabilitation of stroke patients.

With regard to strength and endurance, Dhurva takes a traditional approach. Poses designed to enhance strength and/or endurance are liberally incorporated into a Dhurva practice. The tempo and intensity of a Dhurva session can be modulated to emphasize strength, endurance training, or both. So while sessions can be contemplative and serene, there is flexibility to target increased athleticism as a major practice goal.

DHURVA YOGA

Origins and the Yogistick

Like many modern inventions, Dhurva was not the product of conscious design. It developed mainly through an organic process, the implications of which were not immediately apparent. The roots can be found in my time as a yoga instructor in Southern California where my classes at first were conventional, drawing heavily from Ashtanga and various related forms. Dhurva developed only incrementally; though once the process began, it evolved with surprising speed.

The beginnings were modest enough: In the course of my personal practice I began to use a stick as an aid to stretching. This, in itself, was nothing really new. Athletes who play stick sports such as golf, baseball and cricket routinely use the tools of their trade as a stretching prop. But yoga is not a traditional stick sport and so yoga instructors had not previously made use of this simple device.

Over time, I began to use the stick more and more in my own practice. Because it was so useful in stretching I eventually began to incorporate the stick into my students' lessons. Certain poses which tested range of motion were so obviously advantaged that use of the stick became routine.

But in using the stick so often new uses were quickly discovered — a prop for stretching was not the only possible function. For example, we almost immediately adapted the stick as an aid to balance. As all beginning practitioners know, maintaining balance in, for example, tree pose can be difficult and frustrating. But the stick enabled students to easily find their center of gravity without the problem of falling over. By using the stick as a training tool, they were soon able to hold the pose.

Other uses were developed in due course until the stick became a constant companion to my student yogis.

Ultimately the sticks emerged as a signature feature, differentiating my classes from others. As the classes became more popular, the need for sticks became acute. I therefore began making my own. After a bit of trial-and-error it became clear that wood was the best material, augmented by a rubber cap at each end. With a little more experimentation the optimal size and weight were determined. The Yogistick was born.

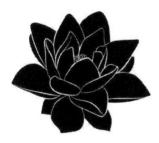

Thus, from a mere prop casually employed in my personal practice, the Yogistick rapidly evolved into a unique and defining feature of my teaching. Curiously, all of this development was natural and intuitive. There was no conscious effort on my part to expand upon use of the stick; its ever-wider role just grew organically from an intrinsic and broad functionality.

It was at this juncture, fostered by comments from my students, that I had an epiphany: The classes which used the stick as a centerpiece really embraced a new and distinctive approach to the yoga experience. Yes, props of various sorts are a common sight in yoga studios. Blocks, for example, are used to assist students in the performance of some poses. In no case, however, is the prop an essential element. Moreover, props are almost always used to support students as they learn traditional poses. The ultimate goal is generally to discard the prop. They are not incorporated into the poses in their final form.

Fully appreciating how the Yogistick had refashioned my teaching, I now focused more consciously upon novel ways to use it. This helped to transform what was originally a glorified form of "yoga with a stick" into a better defined and more formal structure — in short, a thoroughly fleshed out and entirely new style of yoga. At this point, a name for this new approach seemed in order. I chose "Dhurva," which is the Sanskrit word meaning equilibrium.

And so Dhurva came into existence as a distinct entity. While still fitting within the general parameters that define yoga as yoga, Dhurva possesses unique attributes which set it apart. The defining difference, of course, is the Yogistick. But as this volume and others to follow will spell out, there are other nuances as well: in philosophy, in approach, and in teaching methodology.

While Dhurva now represents a complete system for practicing yoga, it continues to evolve. My philosophy is not one restricted by dogma nor limited by past or present practice. Dhurva retains the essentials of traditional yoga, built upon centuries of wisdom and experience. Nevertheless, it represents a significant refinement. In addition, its practice remains open to new knowledge and deeper understanding. Dhurva will continue to develop in the light of continuing experience and novel insight.

I therefore view every class as a means to new knowledge from which Dhurva will evolve. Our practice will continue to build upon historical wisdom while adding its own unique perspective. Like the movements of which it is composed, Dhurva is fluid and dynamic with a form that is ever-changing. This brief summary of the Dhurva story is only the beginning.

Yogistick

First and foremost, the difference between Dhurva and other forms of yoga is the Yogistick. The standard Yogistick is a solid rod or tube, (insert dimensions), with a rubber cup at the end. The Yogistick is deceptive in its simplicity. On first impression, it appears to be just another prop — no different than, say, a block or a strap. But the Yogistick is unique. Unlike blocks or straps which have limited uses, the Yogistick has wide-ranging applications. What follows is a partial catalogue which should give you a sense as to its versatility and the value it adds to the practice of yoga.

The original and most important function of the Yogistick is its use as an aid to stretching. There are several techniques which are suitable to this purpose. For deep stretching, body weight or traction is in some poses not well-suited to optimize the range of motion. Here the Yogistick is put to best effect. A good example is the Miracle I pose, in which the goal is to safely achieve a full range of shoulder extension. Using the body and gravity alone the ideal stretching position is not readily achieved. However, gentle pressure can be exerted through the top of the stick to increase the range of shoulder extension. The pressure can be easily modulated by the yogi so that this is a safe and effective means to enhance the effectiveness of the pose.

In other poses the stick aids stretching by virtue of its weight. The Acceptance pose (known traditionally as the standing forward bend) provides a clear illustration. The extra mass provided by the stick increases traction on the hamstrings and lower back. Here, the downward force added by the Yogistick provides a surprising degree of extra stretch. And if more traction is desired the weight of the Yogistick can be effectively leveraged. Thus, by extending the arm at the shoulder with the stick held by the outstretched hand, tension on a stretched hamstring or other muscle can be significantly increased. This further increases the range of motion.

Other poses also use the weight of the stick to advantage, though in a distinct manner. The quintessential example is Porcupine pose, in which the tendency for students lacking flexibility is to fall over backwards. By holding the stick forward of the center of gravity, this natural tendency is countered so that the posture can be maintained. With practice, flexibility is improved, and the stick becomes unnecessary. But without a counterweight in the early stages of learning, Porcupine pose may present intractable problems. Here the Yogistick makes all the difference.

In other poses the weight of the stick is used as a means to challenge the strength and endurance of the practitioner. A clear example is the side plank, which of course can be done without a prop. But by grasping the stick with the free, elevated hand the degree of difficulty is increased. In this instance the stick is supported by an arm fully extended in the vertical plane and it may appear to add little to the pose. A brief experiment, however, should convince you that the stabilizers in the arm, shoulder and upper back are thoroughly activated when the Yogistick is added. A number of other poses are made more demanding in similar manner.

The Yogistick also provides great advantage in assisting with balance; and this is perhaps its most intuitive function. Of course, humans have for millennia used a walking stick or cane. Its use as an aid to balance is therefore familiar. The only question is why no one thought to use a balancing stick as a yoga prop until now.

In this capacity the stick is especially important as students advance in their practice and begin to attempt more challenging poses. For some of these poses it is difficult or even impossible for newer students to make more than a token attempt without some assistance. In traditional practice a block can sometimes serve this purpose but for most poses the block is too small to be of much use.

The Great Wall pose is illustrative. For advanced practitioners, the stick is not used for balance — full body weight is placed entirely on the grounded foot. But achieving this level of mastery usually takes time. Without the stick, most students will be too unstable to make more than a futile and, ultimately, unproductive attempt. The Yogistick enables even beginning students to work productively on this pose. Still another way in which the Yogistick improves balance involves poses in which the stick itself is balanced. Monkey pose (pictured) and Firefly pose are two good examples. These poses and others test the coordination and kinesthetic sense in a way than traditional poses do not. Unique to Dhurva, they illustrate the power of the Yogistick to expand the horizons of a yoga practice.

Developing a kinesthetic sense — an awareness of how the body is positioned in space — is a goal of traditional yoga practice. A problem arises, however, in that for some poses there is no visual feedback to direct adjustments when positioning is imperfect. In Ostrich pose, for example, the hands are placed behind the back and their precise position is difficult to see. Here the stick provides the means because it indicates the hand position to the yogi by simple reflection in a mirror. If the hands are correctly positioned, the stick can be seen perfectly oriented in the vertical plane. Any displacement to one side or the other indicates a need for repositioning. The length of the stick is a helpful feature here since it amplifies any diversion from the ideal placement of the hands. Thus, even small deviations can be identified and corrected. In other poses as well, the angle assumed by the stick with respect to the body, floor, or side wall provides a ready indicator for orientation of the body in space. As one would suspect, this function assumes special importance during self-practice.

A unique application for the stick is seen in several poses having a purpose to release fascia, the connective tissue that that attaches, stabilizes, encloses, and separates muscles and other internal organs. Here, pressure is exerted by the Yogistick against the body to achieve this effect. The technique duplicates the use of commercially available massage rollers. Both the Fire Log and Impala poses are good examples. Without the stick, fascial release in this manner is not easily accomplished in the normal course of a yoga practice.

In still other poses the stick serves not merely to enhance stretching or facilitate balance or improve strength but as a supporting element integral to the pose. Such poses would be quite impossible without the Yogistick serving as a full structural support. A perfect example is the Black Moon pose, in which the knee and toes of one leg serve as two legs of a tripod while the stick serves as the third. Obviously, such poses are unique to Dhurva.

In much of the foregoing, the utility of the stick is reasonably clear from just looking at someone performing the pose. In others, the value becomes truly clear only with explanation or when one performs the pose oneself. Consider, for example, the Juice pose. You might ask: Why couldn't the pose be done by simply grabbing the feet? And, indeed, it could. But the narrow stick provides a secure structure for the hand to grasp — unlike the foot in which a firm grip is not always so easily maintained. The pose is thus both easier and more effective with the Yogistick than without.

PHILOSOPHY

At first impression, Dhurva may appear as a novelty, differentiated from other forms of yoga only by use of the Yogistick. This characterization, though, is far too narrow. In its development, Dhurva has acquired a unique philosophical framework. As with the physical incidents of practice this framework has evolved over time as my understanding, informed by study and interactions with students and other teachers, has crystalized.

Dhurva ultimately serves as a mechanism to achieve the goals of physical, mental and spiritual well-being. A disciplined and consistent practice will result in high levels of strength, flexibility and stamina. All aspects of health and well-being will be enhanced. Benefit, though, is not limited to the physical. Dhurva will also assist in achieving mental clarity and sharpness of focus. Finally, Dhurva promotes spiritual growth, fostering an internal sense of peace, tranquility and harmony. It is this wide-ranging self-actualization — physical, mental and spiritual — which is the vital purpose of Dhurva practice.

The foregoing perhaps comes as no surprise. These essentials are closely aligned if not identical to the aims of most yoga styles. Yet there are nuances to Dhurva which represent a refinement from traditional teachings. The following short sections address some of the perspectives which inform Dhurvic philosophy. It is not intended as a comprehensive summary but as an introduction which illuminates some important nuances of Dhurvic teachings.

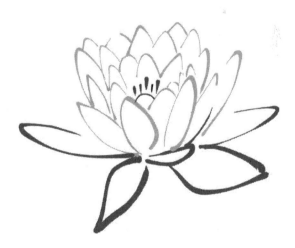

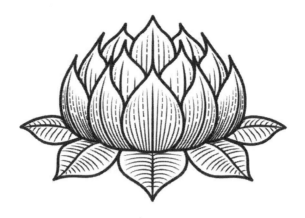

Poses in context

Dhurva, as with any form of yoga, is concerned with the students' ability to correctly perform the poses. However, perfect pose technique is not the ultimate aim of practice. Dhurva, rather, is the means to a far more important end: enhanced physical, mental and spiritual well being outside of the yoga studio. Yes, a dedicated practice will improve one's mastery of the poses, but this ability is a signpost of progress, not an endpoint.

Remember that much of the ability to be proficient with the poses results from factors over which one has no control. Some students will never have the flexibility nor strength to do certain poses. Limitations may be due to genetics, prior injury, or other factors. Many beginning students see this as a failing but such an attitude is rejected by Dhurva. The reasons are twofold. First, since proficiency at the poses is not a primary aim of practice, the inability to perfectly perform one or another pose is hardly of consequence.
Second, Dhurva philosophy holds that we practice maximizing our unique and personal potential, not to achieve some artificial, idealized version of ourselves. The value of yoga, in this view, is found not in achievement relative to an external standard, nor in comparison to the performance of others. A successful Dhurva practice reflects a continual evolution: improved strength and flexibility; a sharper and less encumbered mind; and heightened spiritual awareness, inner peace and harmony. So while the developed ability to perform difficult poses is estimable and useful, such physical skills must be seen in the light of their overall purpose.

Certainly there is satisfaction to be gained in performing difficult poses. And setting one's mind to performing a challenging pose can be a useful motivational device. After all, the benefits of yoga are not always quantifiable or easily demonstrated at a single moment in time. How, for example, could one prove tranquility and inner harmony on demand? Proficiency in performing the poses is therefore a useful proxy for the more profound changes which a dedicated practice will produce. But it is only a proxy and this should not be forgotten. Facility with the poses must be understood in context. Ultimately it is a means and not an end.

Competition

The Dhurvic philosophy is not part of the emerging trend of yoga as a competition sport. I do not offer judgment upon this modern emphasis; it seems to have its place among the many offshoots of traditional practice. But whatever an ultimate judgment, the approach to competitive yoga is very different from that of traditional practice and Dhurva as well. I do not, for example, teach to push through injury or discomfort. Such a "victory" would, in my estimation, be substantially pyrrhic. The Dhurva mentality is not "no pain, no gain."

In short, Dhurva is not a competition. An appreciation for the strength, flexibility, and balance possessed by others is a virtue. Whether you reach such level, though, is largely immaterial. Does this mean that we should take no notice of our peers? Absolutely not. We should be inspired by their accomplishments and strive towards them. When we look at a practitioner who flawlessly executes a difficult pose the attitude engendered should be aspirational, but not because there is any imperative to match them.

The foregoing does not, however, mean that Dhurva approves an attitude of indifference. It is not productive to be satisfied with one's level of achievement in Dhurva. There is always a path to further self-improvement. Engagement with this path is what we seek. It matters little whether you can perform some particular pose or other with perfect form. It only matters that you seek out and travel the path to heightened self-actualization.

The foregoing applies also to the idea that yoga is directed towards the development of a perfect physique. So while a consistent and diligent practice will lead to improvements in one's appearance and can even be a useful adjunct to a program of weight loss, Dhurva yoga is not designed specifically for either body sculpting or weight management. Of course, one might profitably look at the lean and athletic form of someone else in class. But the attitude engendered should be one of admiration without any concurrent sense of self-deprecation or envy. The aims of Dhurva can be achieved without attaining the chiseled look of Greek statuary. One may aspire to achieve an improved physique; but the key is to engage the path towards self-betterment without measuring success or failure with reference to an external standard.

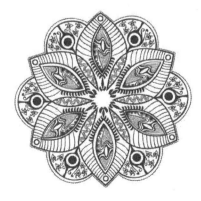

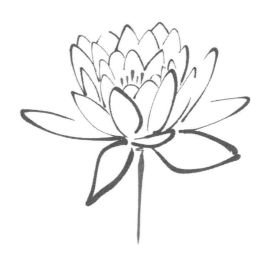

Spirituality

On the spiritual side, Dhurva takes a somewhat different approach than some of the traditional styles of yoga. We do not offer spiritual growth as a mindful product of practicing Dhurva. Thus, our classes are not terribly self conscious with regard to the spiritual side of yoga practice. We do not begin sessions with a Hindi prayer and we do not actively seek transcendental enlightenment. Instead, Dhurva contemplates an organic approach to spiritual growth. We view the spiritual awareness and harmony that yoga engenders as a natural consequence of committed practice. Deepened spirituality emerges as an incident to diligent work in the studio or at home but there are no exercises or poses that are narrowly tailored towards spiritual development.

Thus, finding spiritual virtue through Dhurva is not like a mining operation in which one digs specifically for some valuable commodity. Rather, it is an effect which occurs organically and without special effort. It is similar in this way to good karma, which is achieved not by conduct solely directed towards its capture, but by doing good deeds and performing kindnesses for others. When these things are a daily habit then good karma envelops the individual through a process which is largely unconscious. So it is with the spiritual benefits of yoga; one need not seek them out directly. Spiritual awareness and harmony evolve on their own without being self-consciously pursued. Dhurva is permissive, allowing spiritual growth to occur of its own accord, in concert with the progress of one's yoga practice.

Community

Another feature of Dhurva, though not unique, is its emphasis upon community. Yoga is a multifaceted activity which accommodates many forms and perspectives. These forms coexist in loose association, sharing common elements yet finding diversity in their particulars.

I gratefully acknowledge the foundation which has been laid by yogis in the past. And while I believe that Dhurva offers advantages not found in other forms, this does not represent a disparagement. Each style of yoga has its strengths. All have in common the desire to facilitate self-improvement and self-healing. It is therefore generally true that any yoga is better than no yoga at all. So while I believe that for most practitioners Dhurva will offer specific refinements and benefits, every style of yoga warrants respect. We are part of the greater yoga community and this is an important part of our identity.

In addition to being a part of the global yoga community, Dhurva also creates community at a more local level. While it is possible to take up Dhurva as a solitary endeavor, we strongly encourage practitioners to actively engage with their peers. Share freely your Dhurva experience with others. Teachings spread among students or between instructors inure to the benefit of everyone. The other side of communal practice, of course, is relational. The yoga studio is an ideal venue to meet others and expand one's social circle. Your fellow students and instructors will tend to be like-minded individuals, proactive in the pursuit of both self-improvement and in bettering the world around them. A closer acquaintance with them can be a valuable incident to your study and practice of Dhurva.

Perhaps most valuable in the idea of community is this: As a member of a group that seeks self improvement in cooperation with others, you will be fostering the idea that we are interdependent social beings. The Earth is a small planet on which our health and very survival ultimately depend upon mutual respect, cooperation and support. Establishing and working within an active, socially conscious community is a necessary foundation for harmonious coexistence among the many different races and nations. When practiced as a group endeavor, yoga can be a strong, unifying force for good both locally and around the world. Dhurva therefore incorporates the sense of community as a core feature of its philosophical underpinnings.

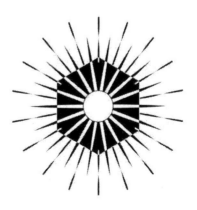

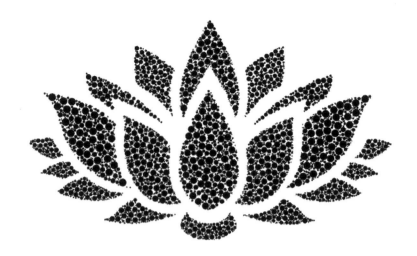

CHAPTER 2
THE PILLARS

YOGA PRACTICE AND STRUCTURE

A yoga class, like most teaching tools, has organization and structure. And like most things with structure, it is built by combining small component elements into a greater, integrated whole. A general process is followed: The smallest, fundamental elements are combined into larger elements which are themselves combined into larger and more complex structures. Ultimately, a relatively small number of moderately complicated elements are joined together, completing the whole.

The process is illustrated by the construction of a house. In the beginning there are only small pieces such as cinder blocks, wooden planks, nails, shingles and the like. These are assembled into higher order structures that comprise modules of construction such as the foundation; the frame; electrical, plumbing and HVAC systems, and so on. These components are tied together to form rooms and connections between them, and the rooms with these connecting elements are in turn combined to create the finished house. As the house is built, higher orders of structure are created and aggregated into a functional whole.

Similarly, a yoga class may be considered in terms of its organization and structure. From this perspective the most fundamental element is the pose. Each pose may be seen as a building block which initially stands in isolation, having on its own a very limited utility. The poses, though, are joined together in a specific sequence. This carefully crafted structure creates a synergy which amplifies the benefit of each individual pose. Properly assembled, the whole becomes much greater than the sum of its parts.

The poses considered individually and in their direct relation to one another, though, does not represent the totality of structure. Just as a house has intermediate layers of structure, so do yoga classes. Most notably, there exists in most yoga classes a tripartite functional structure consisting of a) a warm-up period; b) a working period and; c) a cool-down period. Each of these three elements is comprised of eight to ten individual poses. The warm-up takes place at the beginning of the class and has characteristic features and functions. Poses are chosen to stimulate blood flow, generate body heat, and prepare the body for the more vigorous activity to follow. Movements, for the most part, are minimally demanding of strength and flexibility.

Following the warm up period comes the main body of the class. Here, the demands are greater. Strength, endurance, balance and range of motion are challenged. Mental focus is sharpened. This portion of the class is that in which the student develops the skills which define her practice and from which most of the benefits flow.

Poses at the end of class are chosen to provide a cool down period from the high activity level involved in the middle of the class. During this phase physiological changes are fostered including slowed heart and respiratory rates. Focused attention is replaced by meditative calm. Body and mind are reoriented from the requirements of practice to the demands of life outside of the yoga studio.

Conceptually, we could thus divide all yoga classes into three distinct stages: a warm-up at the beginning; an active phase in the middle; and a cool down period at the end. This division of the yoga class is simple, intuitive and clear to virtually all yoga instructors and students.

Now, if this were the only structure required for a yoga class there would be no necessity for a book about how to sequence poses. But the reality is more complex. Between the foundational elements (the poses) and the broad stages of warm-up, active, and cool down there is an intermediate structure. This consists of small groups of poses which, when placed together sequentially in a class, act as a functional unit. It is this middle range of structure — not as elemental as the poses yet not so broad as the tripartite organization — which is the subject matter of this book. In the jargon of Dhurva Yoga these short sequences are called "pillars."

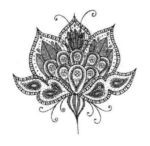

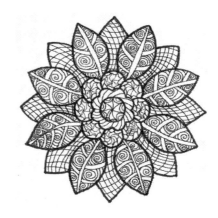

INTRODUCTION TO THE PILLARS

So what, exactly, are the pillars of Dhurva yoga? Simply put, the pillars are short sequences of related poses. They are structured building blocks: more complex than single poses but smaller, simpler and more flexible than the beginning/middle/end structures mentioned in the previous section. Collectively the pillars provide parts from which Dhurva sessions can be logically constructed. Properly used they combine to form a pose sequence that is seamless in continuity, addressed to specific aims, and optimized for safety and effectiveness.

The pillars, though they require some initial work to learn, ultimately ease the task of the instructor or student. Without them, every practice session or class would involve dozens of decisions as to the ordering of poses. The result might not be calamitous but it would be nearly impossible for even the most experienced practitioner or instructor to maximize the benefits of a practice session by making on-the-fly decisions regarding which pose to do next.

There are five pose characteristics which primarily guide pillar design. They are, in no particular order: posture, functionality, fluidity, energy, and balance.
Every pillar embraces at least one of these principles in the assemblage of component poses and most pillars take account of two or more. Each is explained and discussed at some length in the following sections.

VALUE OF THE PILLARS

As a threshold matter it might be asked: Why do we need the pillars? Couldn't one just string poses together one by one? Wouldn't this be adequate to create a yoga class which flowed freely and easily while serving the aims contemplated by the instructor?

Consider again the example of a general contractor tasked with building a home. The contractor could, in theory, just show up at a job site with a truck full of materials and instructions to "build a house." He could then decide where to frame out a room or two; install doors and window frames; and then add a roof in whatever configuration seemed best. And once having these elements in place he could decide where to locate appliances, run plumbing lines, and put in electrical outlets.

Of course, the result would be extremely dysfunctional. A house will be occupied and used. The residents will live in definite patterns of movement and utilization which need to be accommodated by the physical structure. The component parts cannot be placed willy-nilly without producing disharmony. The elements of a house should have a specific relationship one to another within an overall anticipated modus vivendi.

Much better would be to have, at least, rules or guidelines which subserve a general plan. That bedrooms should be clustered together, for example, is a useful guideline that greatly simplifies the overall design. Similarly, understanding the usual flows of traffic will dictate the physical relationship between say, the kitchen and the garage. In short, by understanding how individual parts fit together it becomes much easier to imagine and build out the entire structure.

This necessity for forethought is true not just in house-building but in the building of any complex structure. And since a yoga class is a complex structure, the rule holds here as well. So just as a house can be conceptualized as group of functional elements arranged with specific relationships one to the other, a yoga class can be imagined as a group of individual poses organized into small, functional groupings which are pieced together to form a coherent whole. Individual poses should be organized with attention to the overarching class goals as well as to relationships one-to-another.

In Dhurva, the elemental pieces — the poses — are built into more complex elements — the pillars — which are then linked together to form an entire class. In this way the pillars facilitate the creation of an elegant and functional pose sequence, just as thoughtful design in building construction creates an elegant and functional home.

Thus, the pillars are useful in the original formulation of pose sequences that make up a class. But specific contexts that may require modifying a class also prove their worth. First, classes should be periodically changed up to avoid student boredom or a too casual approach to the practice. When the sequence of a class is exactly the same for weeks or months on end there is a tendency even for diligent students to sometimes just go through the motions, not paying proper attention to breathing or form.

Of course, one could just randomly insert or delete poses but this, in my experience, tends to interfere with the logic of a carefully orchestrated pose sequence. Some poses just don't work well in conjunction with others. Sometimes such unharmonious sequencing can be anticipated while at other times only experience reveals the poor fit. By packaging poses into short, harmonious sequences the pillars can help to ensure a more varied practice while maintaining coherence, continuity and flow.

Second, the composition of classes may change from time-to-time, perhaps even from day-to-day. A class may be comprised of mostly advanced students on one day but have a larger group of intermediate students the next. The instructor will then find it useful to eliminate some poses for a given class while adding others. This can be done pose by pose but the results will tend to be disjointed. The pillars permit the level of difficulty to be easily altered while preserving the logic and harmony of pose sequencing.

Third, within a particular class the instructor may find that a change of plan is in order due to unexpected circumstances. A pre-set program may be rendered undesirable, for example, by a consensus view from the students who wish for an emphasis on core strengthening when the original plan was to focus upon flexibility. To do this pose by pose is difficult even for the most experienced instructor. But by using the pillars, the pace, difficulty or focus of the class can be altered more quickly and easily with minimal concern that poor sequencing will disrupt the flow and energy of the class.

Fourth, it occasionally happens that a class is running substantially behind schedule and is backed up against another class. Or perhaps students are having particular difficulty with one or two particular poses and more than the usual amount of time is devoted to them. It may for these or another reason be useful to eliminate an entire block of poses towards or at the back end of the instruction period. If a class is originally constructed of pillars rather than individual poses, this can be done without disrupting the continuity of the class. Simply drop a pillar (or two) which, as an integrated unit, can be removed completely and without much in the way of mental gymnastics. Such a technique works much better than foregoing individual poses on the fly or abruptly ending class when time for the following class has arrived.

There are, to be sure, other circumstances as well in which the pillars prove to have great practical value. The main point is this: The pillars, once learned and understood, enable the yogi to quickly assemble a pose sequence that comprises a smooth-flowing and functionally coherent class session. They are, in a manner of speaking, a shorthand which expresses years of experience and an evolved logic in creating pose sequences. It is to this logic, the foundation of the pillars, which we now turn our attention.

THE LOGIC OF THE PILLARS

The pillars, as explained in the chapter introduction, are short pose sequences that work harmoniously together. With this in mind one may usefully ask: Why do some poses work well together while others do not? This is an important question whose answer reveals the logic of the pillars.

As it turns out, poses work well — or not so well — with other poses on the basis of just a handful of elements. In this volume we will discuss six of these elements: posture, functionality, energy, balance, difficulty and fluidity.

Some of these elements are simply characteristics of the poses which may be in common or different between any pair. For example, a pose may be a tranquil setting for meditation or, alternatively, a robust physical challenge. Another pose may be well-matched or not on the basis of this quality alone. If an instructor wishes to lead a quiet, contemplative class she will bundle poses which are serene and physically undemanding. Conversely, if the emphasis is on some aspect of physical conditioning then calming poses would not be part of the pillars employed.

The foregoing may suggest that bundling poses into a pillar is rather simple. Unfortunately, this is not the case. The interplay between poses may be nuanced and subtle. Simply choosing poses with a common characteristic is for that reason a generally ineffective approach to pillar construction. We will discuss the fine points that govern pillar construction in a later section. But to begin, the following short sections will acquaint you with the conceptual building blocks from which the pillars are crafted.

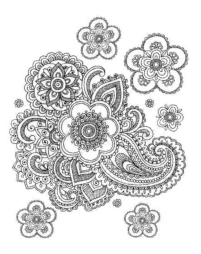

Posture

Yoga poses can be categorized by the dominant posture of the body maintained during the pose. The possibilities include standing, sitting, kneeling, lying prone, lying supine, and crouching. It is axiomatic in yoga that poses having the same dominant posture will tend to work well together in a sequence.

Posture, however, is never alone an adequate basis for grouping poses in a short sequence. Simply because two poses are performed in the standing position, for example, does not mean that they belong in the same pillar. Conversely, there are poses which employ different postures, e.g., standing and sitting, which flow without effort, one into the next.

Identity of posture is thus a useful factor in pairing poses within a single pillar but is not an absolute. So while identity of posture is often a starting point for pillar construction, the creation of pillars is a more nuanced exercise that requires consideration of all six principles of construction.

Functionality

Frequently, poses are linked by a common emphasis upon some particular physiological function. Thus, for example, a short sequence of poses may target core strength, or hip flexibility, or balance.

The function referred to here may mean one of several things. It may refer to the strengthening of a specific muscle group or related set of muscle groups. A specific pillar may therefore be designed to target, for example, core strength or strength of the axial skeleton. Alternatively, function here may refer to the range of motion in one or several body parts. Yet it may have a broader meaning which could include attention to the mental side of practice; or cardiovascular conditioning. A pillar may address any one of these functions and sometimes multiple functions simultaneously.

Many if not most of the pillars are themed with some element of functionality. Therefore the poses comprising a particular pillar will frequently target a specific function. When several of these pillars are used in succession the class taken as a whole will have the specific, functional focus.

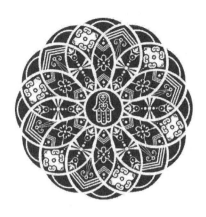

Energy

As I have discussed above, yoga classes tend to take on the collective energy level of its students; and this may create a challenge for the instructor. As experienced yoga instructors know, students come to class with moods that reflect their daytime experiences. Not infrequently this will work at cross purposes to the intentions of the instructor. A class planned to be meditative and serene may be peopled by highly animated students primed for a challenging workout. Or, at the other end of the spectrum, a class designed to be physically and mentally demanding may find a group of students who are somewhat lethargic and disengaged. The dominating mood may be due to the weather, news of the day, or anything at all. But whatever the cause, the instructor must respond appropriately or the session will be frustrating and unproductive.

By controlling activity levels the instructor can moderate the overall mood and focus of the students. Thus, if a class initially is sluggish and the students inattentive, the instructor can gradually ramp up the energy level with pillars designed for that purpose. Conversely, when the students come to class a bit unfocused and hyperactive, the instructor may wish to create, at least temporarily, a quieter and more subdued mood from which attention may be refocused.

When students are not properly primed for the planned work the instructor can use appropriate pillars to reset the mood. Only then can the work designated for the class begin in earnest. Thus, a subset of the pillars are created to either elevate or temper the energy level of the class. They may be used to either set a tone for an entire class or cause the overall energy levels to wax and wane as the class moves from start to finish.

Balance

A key concept in yoga is balance. This is a word with a rich set of meanings, any or all of which may apply in a specific context. With reference to a specific pose it may mean the neuromuscular tools needed to stay upright. With reference to the broad aims of a yoga practice it may mean the weighted attention to physical, mental and spiritual well-being. For purposes of this section, however, we mean something else: the need to maintain strength and flexibility in opposing muscles and joints of the body as well as symmetry between the right and left sides.

Attention to this meaning of balance can be found in multiple pillars. Perhaps most important, poses must include movement in forward flexion as well as extension. We can see this clearly in relation to those poses that involve forward bending and stretching. Such poses should, in most or all cases, be followed immediately or shortly thereafter by poses in which a counter-movement occurs. A number of pillars for this reason incorporate a movement of forward flexion followed by a movement involving whole-body extension. A good example is found in pillars which include both cat and cow poses, performed in alternating sequence. Of course, these balancing movements need not always be done in rapid succession. Nevertheless, it is frequently advantageous to perform the counter movements immediately and some of the pillars are designed with this in mind.

This particular concept of balance also applies to poses designed to strengthen one group of muscles working in a single plane across a joint. A pose which strongly utilizes the biceps muscle, for example, results in flexion at the elbow. The principle of balance therefore offers that the day's practice also include extension at the elbow which employs the triceps muscle. Similarly, a pose that produces abduction at the hip (moving the legs apart) may benefit most if the contrary movement of adduction (moving the legs together) also be done. The pillars take full account of this necessity and are sequenced accordingly.

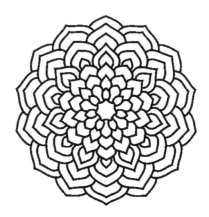

Difficulty

That degree of difficulty is important in pose sequencing should occasion no surprise. Obviously there are limits to the extent that challenging poses can be performed sequentially. At the same time, the use of long sequences which include only elementary poses would clearly not be suitable, save in a beginner's class. Thus, degree of difficulty is often characterized by a carefully orchestrated ebb and flow, the specifics of which require experience and judgment to manage successfully.

The foregoing properly suggests that manipulating difficulty within a class structure is a complex task. There are no simple and general rules which can serve as a reliable guide. Sometimes difficult poses can be sequenced back-to-back (or even back-to-back-to-back) while at other times even two difficult poses in sequence would be problematic. Sequencing poses to properly manage degree of difficulty demands experience. Without such experience it is no easy matter to design a class that is both effective and safe.

Fluidity

One element that is superimposed upon virtually all of the pillars is something without a familiar descriptive term. I will use here the term "fluidity," which seems to capture the essence of it. Fluidity, as the common meaning would suggest, describes the way in which one pose flows into the next.

When fluidity is properly incorporated into a pillar, poses flow seamlessly one into the other. To the greatest extent possible one pose should transition smoothly to the next, without the need for awkward readjustments of posture, inefficient handling of the Yogistick, or ungainly movement.

The entire pillar, taken as a whole, should have a choreographed feel to the practitioner. This is not, however, the same as choreography as used in performance dancing. How the sequence of yoga poses looks to an outside observer is not important; yoga is not an exercise in aesthetics. Movements are choreographed for the benefit of the student, not some imaginary audience.

Pillars are never constructed solely for the purpose of emphasizing fluidity. In this way fluidity differs from the other organizing principles which may be the primary basis for pillar structure. Fluidity is a consideration in every pillar, so that certain poses are combined preferentially with certain others; and particular poses are linked to other poses in a particular sequence. Conversely, those poses which do not flow smoothly, one into the other, are rarely if ever incorporated as successive elements in a single pillar.

HOW TO USE THIS BOOK

The sudden introduction to a large number of pillars may seem daunting. And perhaps it should be if the goal were to simply memorize them. But I am not recommending that approach.

While in a perfect world it would be best to know all of the pillars, as a practical matter this is not necessary. The key is to quickly master those pillars which have frequent application in your practice or classes. Further learning can then gradually proceed from that knowledge base.

So how to begin? Initially, one should read the textual material in this volume and understand the basic principles which direct pillar construction. This is essential. Once these principles are thoroughly understood then learning the pillars will be easier since their underlying logic will be clear. And your use of them will become more than just an unthinking, mechanical process.

Next, take some time to casually flip through the book. Find those poses which you use most often or which you would like to incorporate into your classes or personal practice. Pillars which contain those poses will be most useful and should be learned first. Once those pillars are mastered, broader and more in depth study is in order — but this can be done over an extended period of time and in accord with your specific requirements. Always, the emphasis should be upon utility rather than complete and perfect knowledge. Dhurva is a practical art, not an exercise in academics.

Finally, experienced teachers may find it useful to experiment. Remember, Dhurva is not static. Use the foundational principles articulated in this volume but continue to find new ways that the Yogistick can add to the yoga experience. And when you have new ideas, share them with the Dhurva community. Our collective wisdom is far greater than that of any individual. I welcome new insights and am grateful to my students who seem to teach me as much as I teach them.

NUANCES OF PILLAR CONSTRUCTION

Thus far, we have outlined the pose features which form the basis for pillar construction. In a single pillar, all of the poses will share commonality in at least one of the aforementioned categories — posture, fluidity, functionality, difficulty, balance, or energy.

Of course, any two poses are likely to be similar in regard to at least one of the categories. This does not necessarily mean that they are good candidates to be included in a single pillar. Conversely, few poses are identical to another with respect to all of the enumerated categories. When two poses are compatible in some ways but poorly compatible in others as is typically the case, only judgment and experience will establish which factor(s) are most important. The ultimate judgment as to suitability for inclusion in a single pillar is therefore determined on the basis of such judgment and experience.

For example, just because two poses share a similar or identical posture does not guarantee that they will work well together. The pose pair of Horse twist/Evolved star, illustrates the problem. Both employ a wide, standing base with knees bent and toes angled outward. The two poses, in appearance, therefore seem a natural fit.

In fact, Horse twist and Evolved star would be poor partners. The two poses produce considerable stress upon the lower back, an anatomically vulnerable area. So while yoga in general and Dhurva in particular targets the lower back, such attention is exercised with caution. Poses which make demands upon the lumbar spine should not, as a rule, be done sequentially. At a minimum there should be an intervening pose which momentarily relieves the stress and provides a safe haven between the two.

The same consideration governs the recommendation against using Ostrich pose and Half Lift pose together. Although they do share common elements and a transition from one to the other can be accomplished smoothly, both make significant demands upon the lower back. They are best performed as components of different pillars, with care taken that they are not joined in direct sequence when different pillars containing each are employed sequentially.

Just as some poses which intuitively seem to go together are best done apart, some pose pairs which seem a poor fit may actually work well in tandem. A useful illustration is the combination of Fish pose and Monkey pose. These two poses are very different in most of the features which we have previously claimed as the basis for pose pairing. Fish pose involves a pronounced arch of the back while Monkey pose involves forward flexion. Moreover, the very different positions of the stick would seem to make a smooth transition somewhat awkward. Fish pose emphasizes stretch in extension combined with strength while Monkey pose is less demanding of strength but more demanding of balance.

Despite these differences, however, these two poses are well paired. In fact, the difference in position of the spine constitutes the foundation for using these poses in a single pillar. The fundamental aspect of Fish pose, extension of the entire spine, is gently counteracted by Monkey pose. The anatomic relationships are not entirely dissimilar to the familiar sequencing of Cat and Cow poses which together combine as a very useful stretch-counter stretch pairing. The other differences between Fish pose and Monkey pose are not so important here and can safely be ignored; and the transition from Fish pose to Monkey pose is less awkward than at first appears. Of course, this beneficial sequencing relationship is not immediately apparent. Only years of experience and much trial-and-error demonstrated the value in using these poses together.

Another example is the pose pairing of Xena Warrior and Eagle. Visually and functionally, the two poses appear very different. Xena Warrior is supported by a lunge position while Eagle pose involves balancing on a single leg. On casual inspection there is little which seems to connect them. But in this instance the fluid transition possible from Xena Warrior pose to Eagle pose is the dominant consideration. Also, the shift takes the heavy burden from the right leg in Xena Warrior pose and replaces it with more modest — but still significant — workload of the single leg stance. Thus, the two poses work well in conjunction though intuition would not immediately label them as a useful pairing.

When difficulty is due to problems with balance, however, one should generally not be aggressive in sequencing the poses serially. Only the most advanced students will, as a rule, be able to maintain the focus required to perform three or more poses which make strong demands upon balance. Nor should poses demanding large expenditures of energy generally be performed immediately prior to poses which severely challenge balance. In those instances, strength should be preserved so that the focus can be on balancing, rather than marshaling the power which may be a pose requirement.

The foregoing, of course, is not a comprehensive guide to pillar construction. Taken together, however, these examples teach a valuable lesson: Pillars are not built upon casual inspection. Only due care and consideration informed by years of experience enable pillars to be advantageously constructed. The pillars collected in this volume have received the requisite time and attention, and will provide the basis for sequencing poses for your classes and personal practices no matter the focus or demand characteristics of a given circumstance.

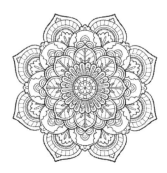

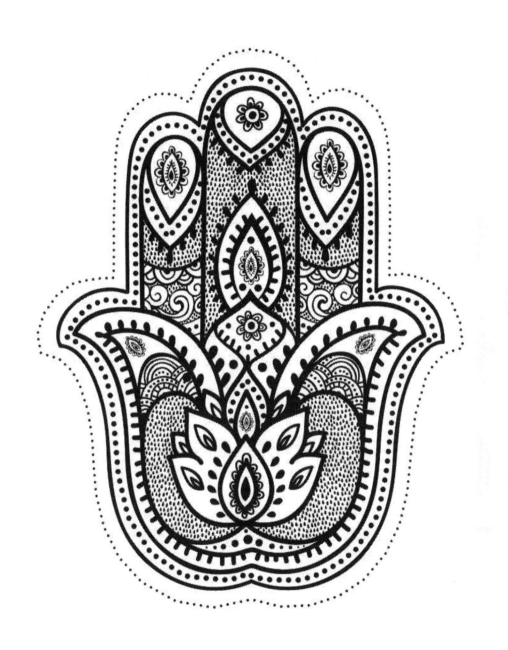

Pillar Pose and Sequence Combinations

Floor

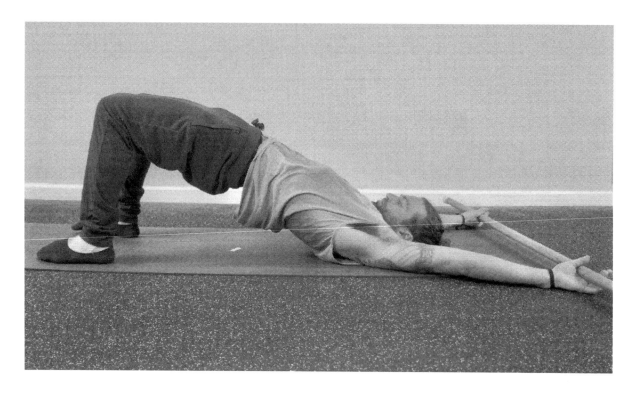

Pillar: Floor
Pose: Bridge
Benefits: • Opens the chest, heart, and shoulders • Stretches the spine, the back of the neck, the thighs, and the hip flexors •
Tips: *Use your butt muscles, thighs and tailbone to tilt the pelvis. Pull your tail up between your legs.*

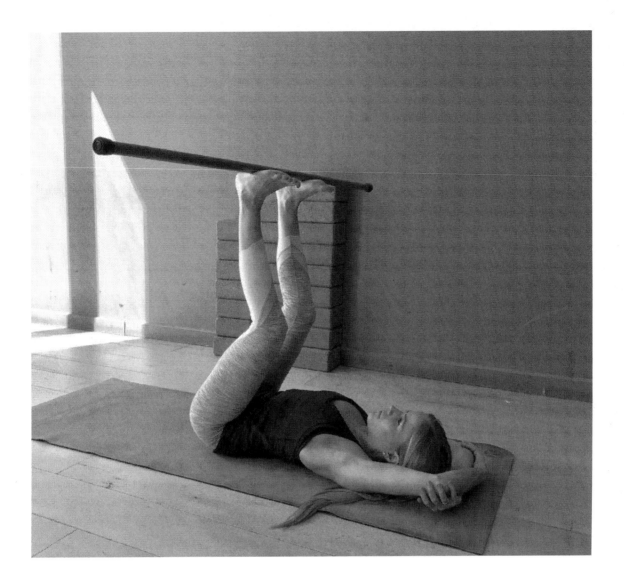

Pillar: Floor
Pose: Monkey
Benefits: • Elevating the legs promotes drainage from excess fluid build-up • Increased circulation of blood back to the heart • Reduces swelling and pain in the lower extremities • Reduces the curve of the lumbar spine, which elongates and stretches the back muscles • Strengthens the core •
Tips: *Patience is key. Lengthen your spine.*

Sitting

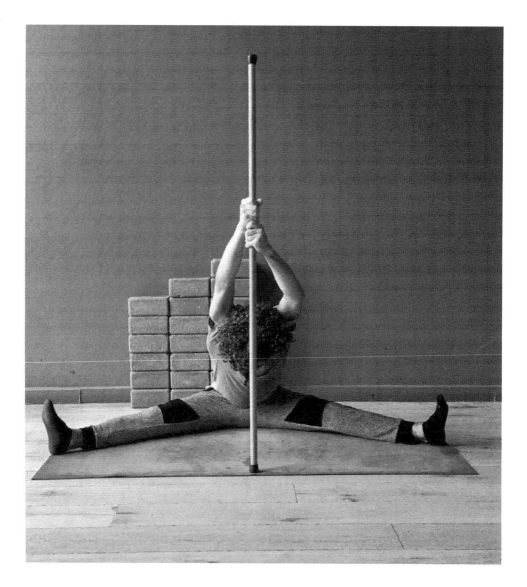

Pillar: Sitting
Pose: Miracle III
Benefit: • Stretches the insides and backs of the legs • Strengthens the spine • Releases groins • Promotes opening in the scapula and increases circulation in the head, neck and shoulders •
Tips: *Flex your toes in and scoot your pelvis forward. Loose head, neck and shoulders.*

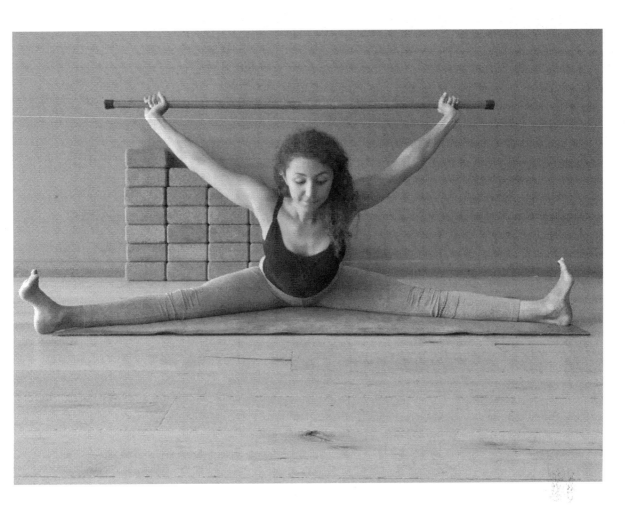

Pillar: Sitting
Pose: Axis
Benefits: • Stretches the insides and backs of the legs • Strengthens the core and spine • Focuses the mind • Releases groins • Promotes opening in the scapula and increases circulation in the head, neck and shoulders •
Tips: *Lead with your belly and tilt your chest up.*

Kneeling

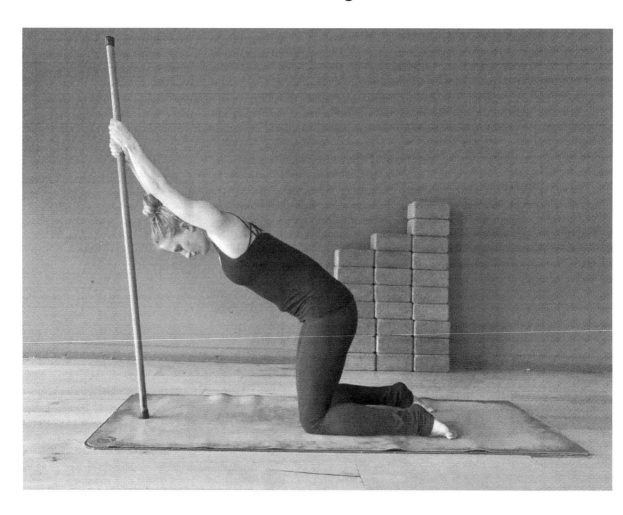

Pillar: Kneeling
Pose: Miracle II
Benefits: • Activates stomach muscles • Strengthens the spine • Promotes opening in the scapula and increases circulation in the head, neck and shoulders •
Tips: *Strong hands, heavy tailbone, loose head, neck and shoulders.*

Triangle

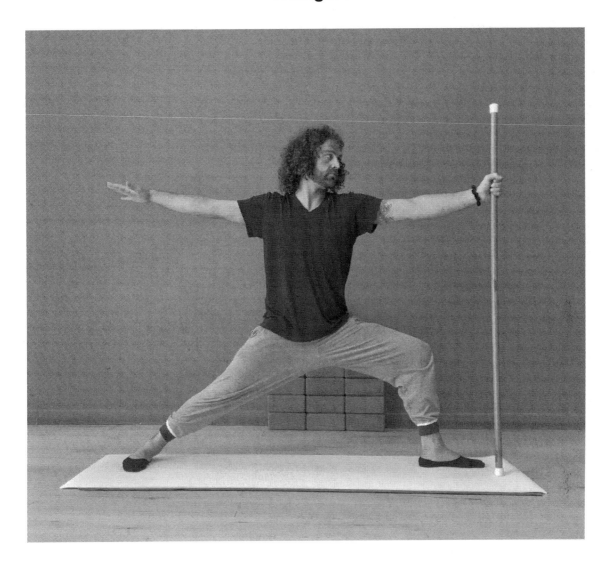

Pillar: Triangle

Pose: Warrior II

Benefits: • Strengthens the legs • Opens the hips and chest • Develops concentration, balance and groundedness • Improves circulation and respiration • Energizes the entire body •

Tips: *Keep you hands up and parallel your waist to the floor. Thighs rotate in and up.*

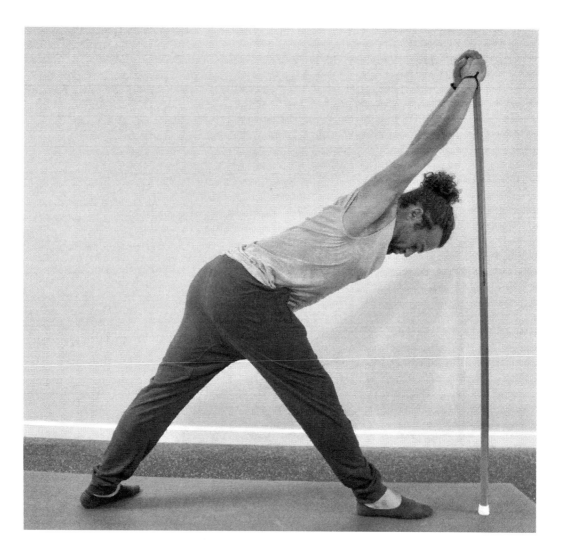

Pillar: Triangle
Pose: Miracle V
Benefits: • Stretches the spine • Strengthens the legs and spine • Promotes opening in the scapula and increases circulation in the head, neck and shoulders •
Tips: *Strong hands, firm legs and square your hips.*

Belly

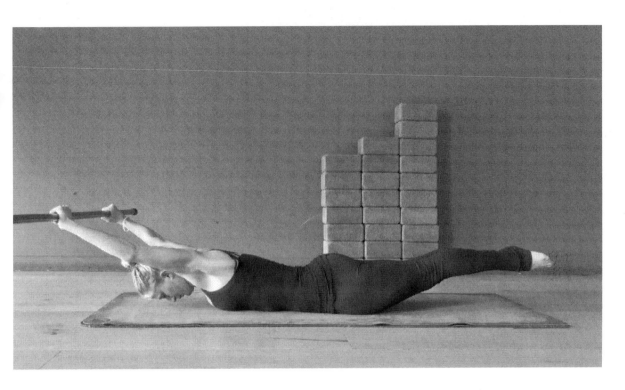

Pillar: Belly
Pose: Magnetic Field
Benefits: • Stretches and strengthens your chest, shoulders, arms, legs, and glutes •
Keeps your back flexible • Improves your circulation •
Tips: *Biceps to ears and point your toes. Super long arms! Tilt pelvis down.*

Standing

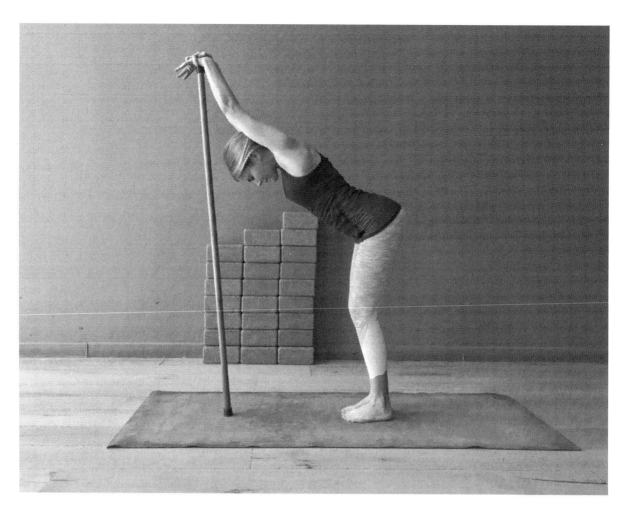

Pillar: Standing
Pose: Miracle I
Benefits: • Decompresses your spine which decreases risk of back injury and helps correct posture • Increases grip strength • Increases core stability •
Tips: *Long arms and straight legs. Strength restorative.*

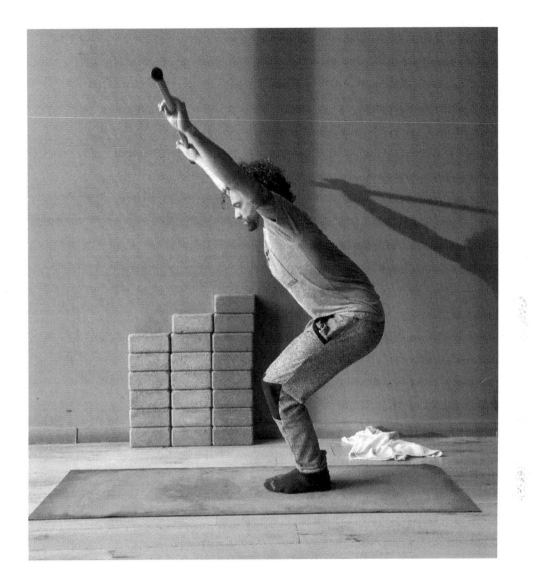

Pillar: Standing
Pose: Chair
Benefits: • Tones leg muscles excellently • Strengthens hip flexors, ankles, calves, and back • Stretches chest and shoulders • Strengthens the core •
Tips: *Arms in line with ears. Grab the floor with your feet.*

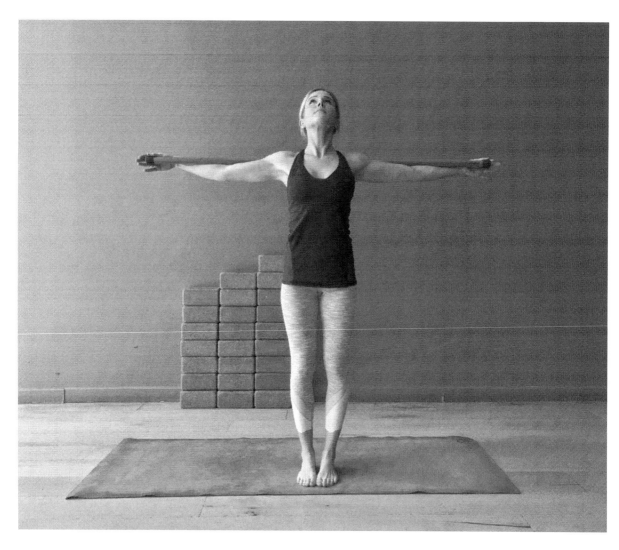

Pillar: Standing
Pose: Quick
Benefits: • Improves posture • Strengthens thighs, knees, and ankles • Steadies breathing • Increases strength, power, and mobility in the feet, legs, and hips • Firms abdomen and buttocks •
Tips: *Light feet, stand tall and challenge wingspan.*

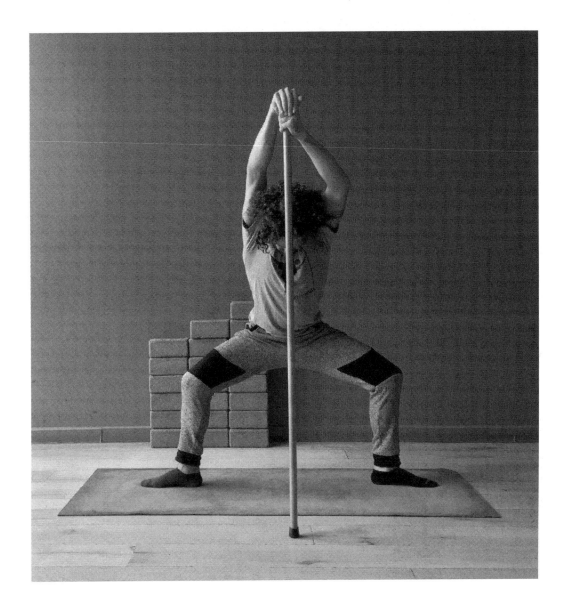

Pillar: Standing
Pose: Miracle VI
Benefits: • Strengthens the core and leg muscles • Teaches balance • Sets a strong foundation for the entire practice • Builds heat in the body • Opens the ankles, knees and hips •
Tips: *Hands up, toes out, strong tummy, firm legs.*

Lunge

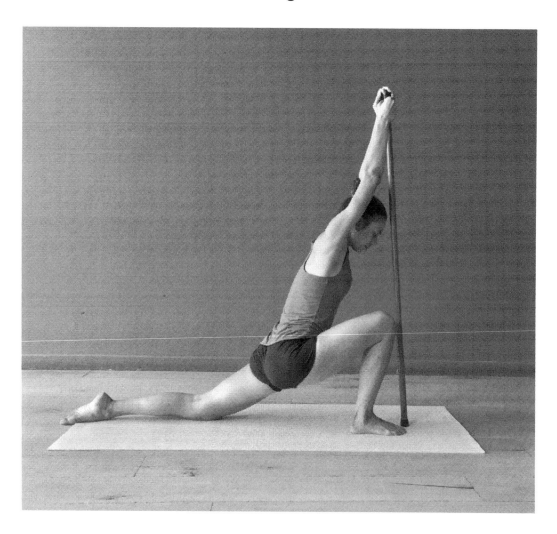

Pillar: Lunge
Pose: Miracle IV
Benefits: • Releases tension in your hips • Stretches your hamstrings, quads, and groin • Strengthens your knees • Strengthens the core • Promotes opening in the scapula and increases circulation in the head, neck and shoulders •
Tips: *Strong hands, hip flexor forward and down, relax your head, neck and shoulders.*

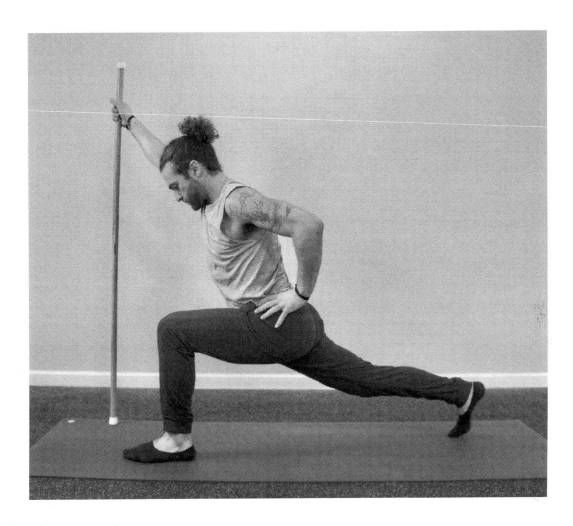

Pillar: Lunge
Pose: Capricorn
Benefits: • Opens your groins and hips • Stretches and tones your legs, especially thighs • Strengthens your knees, ankles and waist • Lengthens the spine, thereby stretching the chest •
Tips: *Firm up butt, legs and core. Light back foot, strong front leg. Always breathing.*

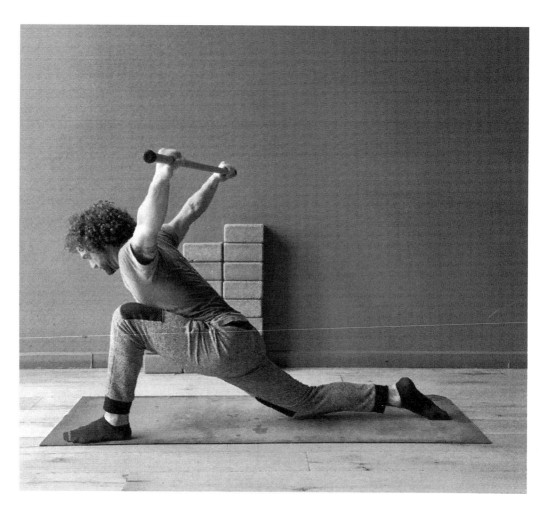

Pillar: Lunge
Pose: Low Lunge
Benefits: • Releases tension in your hips • Stretches your hamstrings, quads, and groin • Strengthens your knees • Helps build mental focus • Strengthens the core • Promotes opening in the scapula and increases circulation in the head, neck and shoulders •
Tips: *Hips forward and down. Strong core. Stay committed. Untuck back toes.*

Balancing

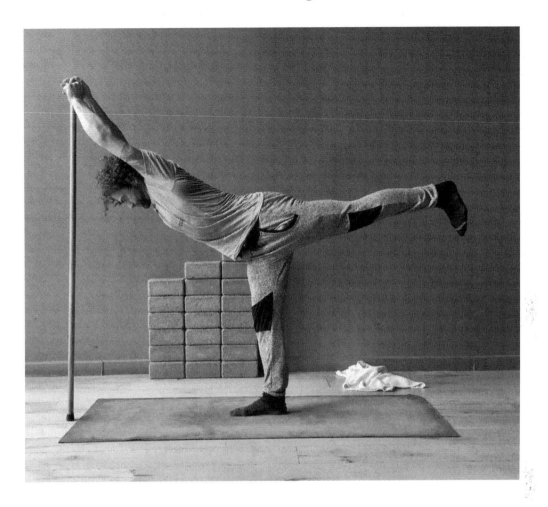

Pillar: Balancing
Pose: Balancing Stick
Benefits: • Strengthens the arms, upper thighs, buttocks and hips • Helps to relieve stress from the spine • Helps to prevent varicose veins • Strengthens the core •
Tips: *Square pelvis and chest to floor. Take up lots of space above your mat. Patience. Tug of war at your belly button.*

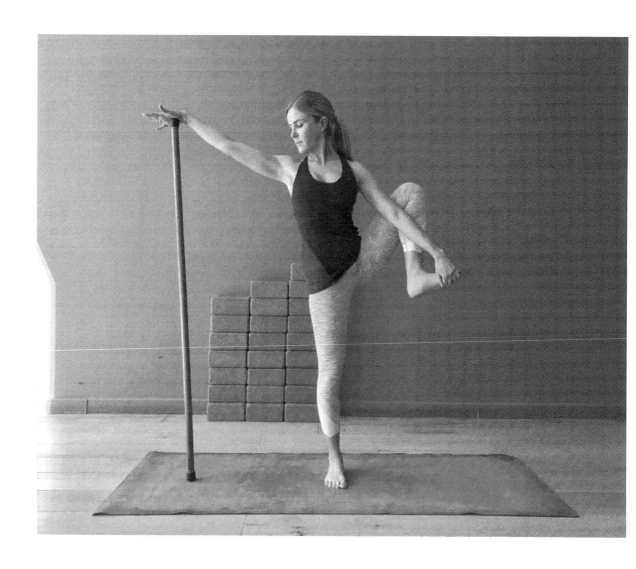

Pillar: Balancing
Pose: Gratitude
Benefits: • Strengthens the legs and ankles • Stretches the backs of the legs •
Improves sense of balance •
Tips: *Hips forward. Stand tall and focus your sight.*

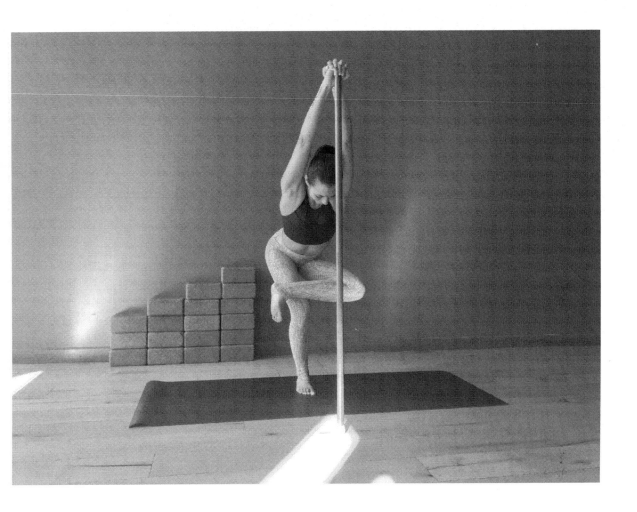

Pillar: Balancing
Pose: Humble Gypsy
Benefits: • Strengthen quadriceps, ankle and foot muscles • Tones the core • Stretches the outer hip and glute muscles • Relieves lower back tension •
Tips: *Bend your standing leg! Firm legs and use your core. Flex floating toes inward.*

Arm Balance

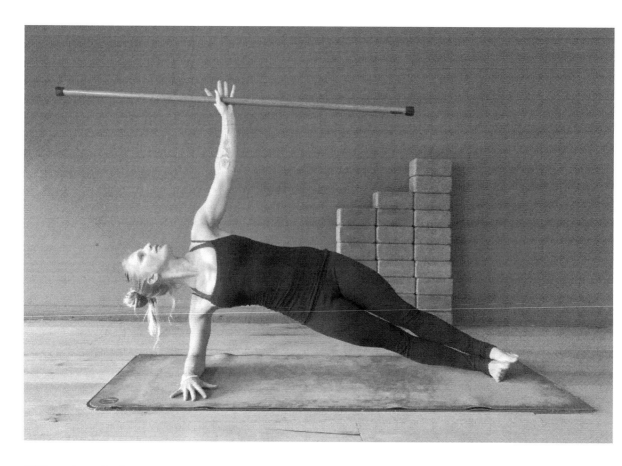

Pillar: Arm Balance
Pose: Forearm Side Plank
Benefits: • Tones your forearms, upper arms, shoulders, and spine • Strengthens muscles around the spine • Improves posture • Sculpts the abdominal muscles • Improves balance, concentration, and focus •
Tips: *Use your whole body! Hips in line with head and ankles. Take up space. Palm the floor from fingers to elbow.*

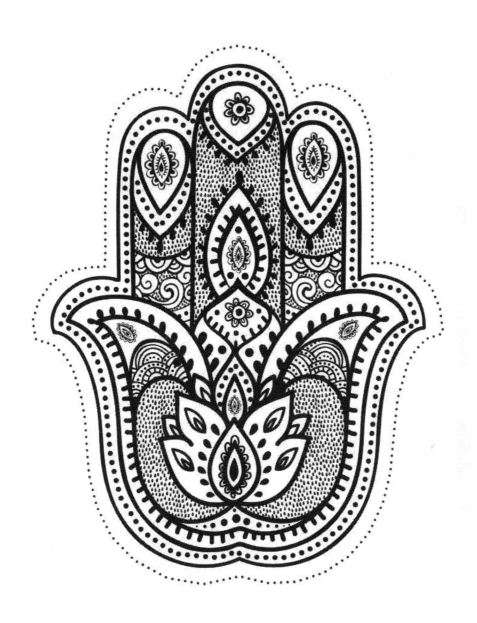

Pillar Sequences
Floor

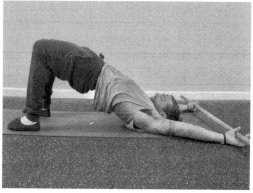

Bridge

3 times, 5 - 10 deep breaths

Tip: Grab the floor with your feet. Toes, knees, hips, shoulders aligned. Strong core and pelvis.

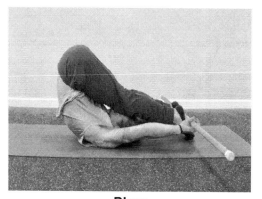

Plow

3 times, 5 deep breaths

Tip: Breathing here is everything. Stay longer and reap the benefits.

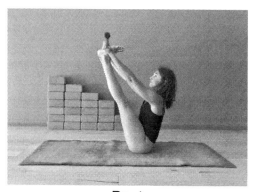

Boat

3 times, 5 - 10 deep breaths

Tip: Light hands and feet. All stomach strength. Move shoulders downward.

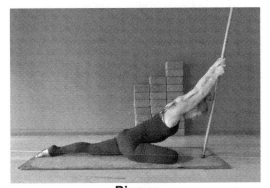

Pigeon

1 minute both sides

Tip: Hands up and both hips toward the floor. Keep your head centered. Breathe it out.

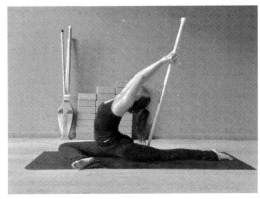

Deep Pockets

5 - 10 deep breaths on each side

Tip: Hands up and pivot your stick close to your body. Be warmed up.

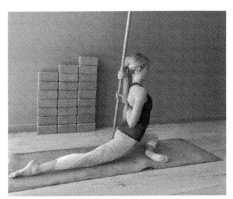

Comet

5 - 10 deep breaths on each side

Tip: Strong tummy and stay balanced. Move elbows inward towards the body. Less is more.

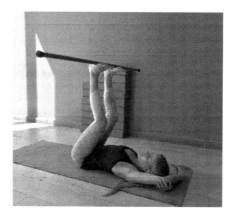

Monkey
Hold for 1 minute and switch grip
Tip: Tailbone slightly off the floor. Bend your knees and practice patience.

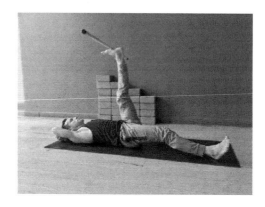

Lame Duck
45 - 60 seconds both sides and switch elbow / forearm grip
Tip: Eye focus and bouyancy are essential. Walk out extending leg.

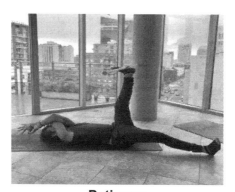

Patience
45 - 60 seconds both sides and switch eagle arm grip
Tip: Long spine from neck to tailbone. Eagle arms way up. Fingers toward the floor.

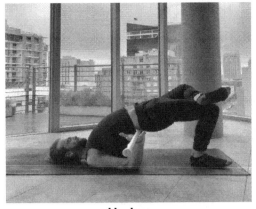

Umbra

5 - 10 deep breaths on each side

Tip: Think strength and restorative. Parallel hips to floor.

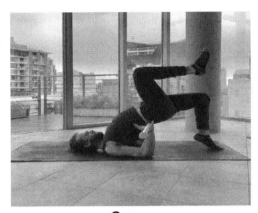

Gypsy

5 - 10 deep breaths on each side

Tip: Tip toes of standing foot. More strength needed than you think.

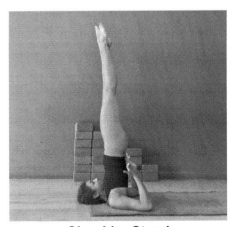

Shoulder Stand

10 breaths

Tip: Use stick to angle pelvis over shoulders. Point toes and press feet away from face.

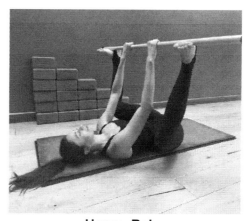

Happy Baby

5 - 10 deep breaths rocking on each side

Tip: Light hands and feet. Use stick to slide feet out.Frame your space.

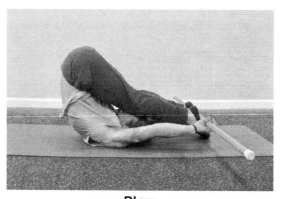

Plow

3 times, 5 -10 deep breaths

Tip: Breathing here is everything. Stay longer and reap the benefits.

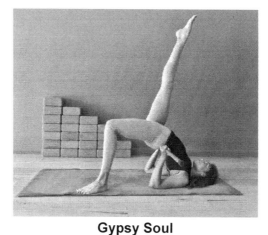

Gypsy Soul

5 - 10 deep breaths on each side

Tip: The Yogistick is just an assist. Stay strong in standing leg.

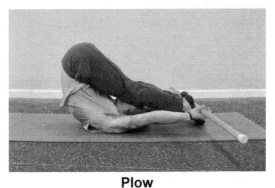

Plow
3 times, 5 deep breaths
Tip: Breathing here is everything. Stay longer and reap the benefits.

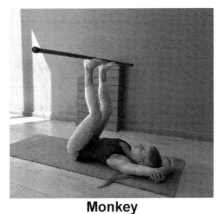

Monkey
Hold for 1 minute and switch grip
Tip: Tailbone slightly off the floor. Bend your knees and practice patience.

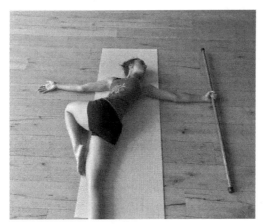

Terrain Twist
25 seconds both sides
Tip: Use YogiStick as a weight. Relax body similar to receiving a massage.

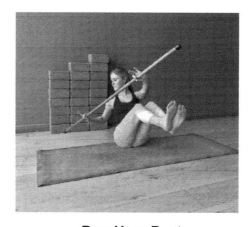

Row Your Boat

5 - 10 deep breaths on each side

Tip: Heavy tailbone and strong stomach. Hips stay forward and use your legs

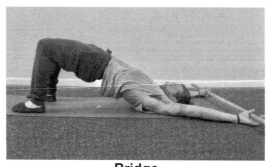

Bridge

3 times 5 - 10 deep breaths

Tip: Grab the floor with your feet. Toes, knees, hips, shoulders aligned. Strong core and pelvis.

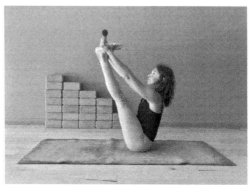

Boat

3 times 5 - 10 deep breaths

Tip: Light hands and feet. All stomach strength. Lighten shoulders downward.

Sitting

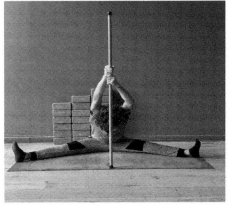

Miracle III

I minute with each hand on top

Tip: Hands up and pivot top of stick away from you. Strong hands and tummy. Relax your head and toes.

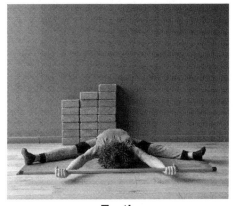

Earth

10 deep breaths

Tip: Reverse grip and lead with your chest. Patience and consistency.

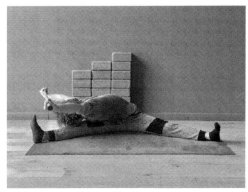

Xian

5 - 10 deep breaths on each side

Tip: Reverse grip and lead with your chest. Inside shoulder towards outside shin.

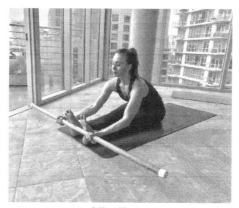

Yin Fold

10 deep breaths

Tip: Light hands and feet. Heels away from you. Widen hands to customize stretch.

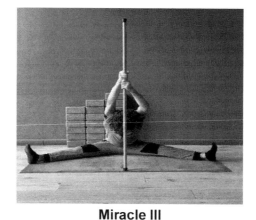

Miracle III

I minute with each hand on top

Tip: Hands up and pivot top of stick away from you. Strong hands and tummy. Relax your head and toes.

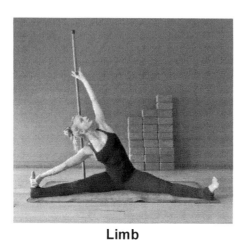

Limb

10 deep breaths on each side

Tip: Pivot stick near outside hip and walk stretching arm way up. Flex your tummy. Long limbs.

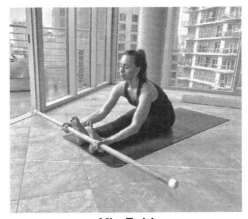

Yin Fold

10 deep breaths

Tip: Light hands and feet. Heels away from you. Widen hands to customize stretch.

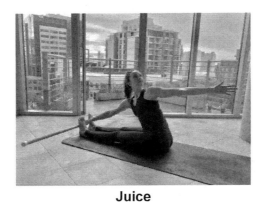

Juice

5 - 10 deep breaths on each side

Tip: Strong inside, light twist. Grab Yogistick with light energy. Keep hips square forward.

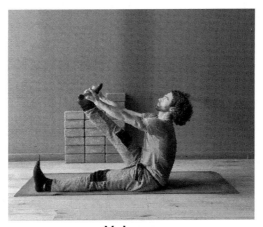

Volcano

5 deep breaths on each side

Tip: Light hands and feet. Bicep grip and grow slowly. Keep hips square.

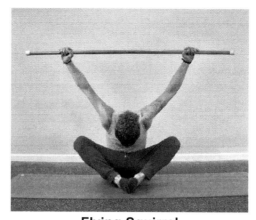

Flying Squirrel
5-10 deep breaths
Tip: Prayer your feet and press together with strength. Light body. Chest forward.

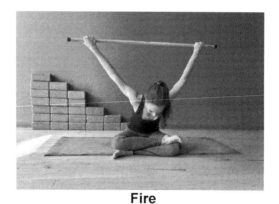

Fire
30 - 45 seconds with each leg on top
Tip: Stack your shins as best as possible. Strong core with light sit bones. Reverse grip.

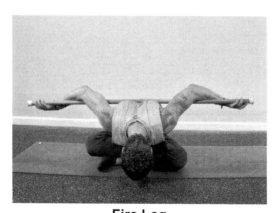

Fire Log
5 -10 deep breaths on each side
Tip: Wrap your fingers around the stick and hold. Think heart to shins. Big deep breaths.

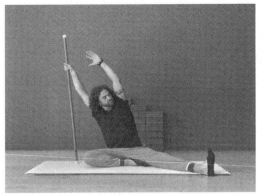

Wind

10 deep breaths on each side

Tip: Seal back of your legs to the ground. Pivot the Yogistick close to hip and keep arms lifted.

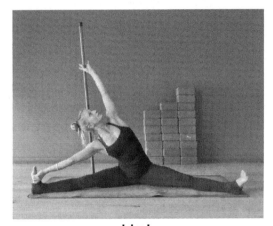

Limb

10 deep breaths on each side

Tip: Pivot stick near outside hip and walk stretching arm way up. Flex your tummy. Long limbs.

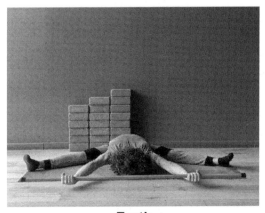

Earth

10 deep breaths

Tip: Reverse grip and lead with your chest. Patience and consistency.

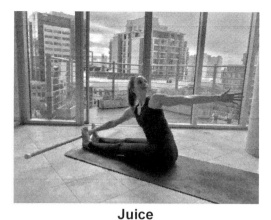

Juice

5 -10 deep breaths on each side

Tip: Strong inside, light twist. Grab YogiStick with strength. Keep hips square forward.

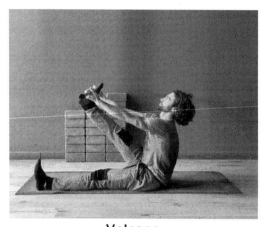

Volcano

5 deep breaths on each side

Tip: Light hands and feet. Bicep grip and grow slowly. Keep hips square.

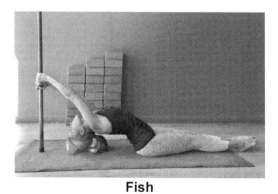

Fish

30 - 45 seconds with each hand on top

Tip: Less is more here. Create space to release your head back between your arms.

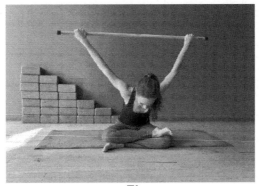

Fire

30 - 45 seconds with each leg on top

Tip: Stack your shins as best as possible. Strong core with light sit bones. Reverse grip.

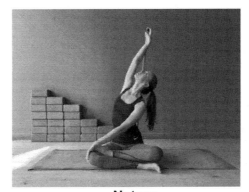

Nature

5 - 10 deep breaths on each side

Tip: Stack shins as best as possible. Use hand on knee to twist upward. Top hand way up.

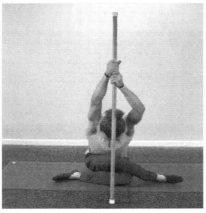

Pulsar

10 deep breaths on each side

Tip: Stack knees on top of each other. Sit bones down. Chin towards your knees. Hands up.

Kneeling

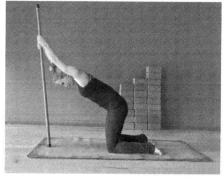

Miracle II
30 - 45 seconds with each hand on top
Tip: Squeeze imaginary block between legs. Relax head and shoulders. Hands up on stick.

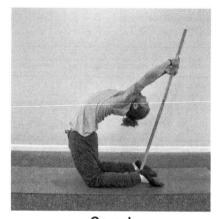

Camel
5 - 10 deep breaths with each hand on top
Tip: Start easy. Create space for your head. Heart over knees. Hands way up. Less is more.

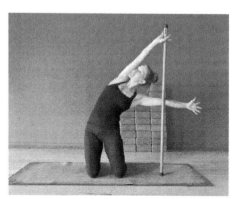

Seahorse
5 - 10 deep breaths on each side
Tip: Both knees and stick aligned on floor. Extend arms up and out. Dynamic hands.

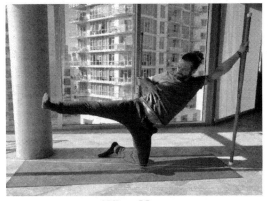

Wise Man

5 deep breaths on each side

Tip: Stack hips and grounded knee. Stick and knee alignment. Spread stick arm, body and extend leg out.

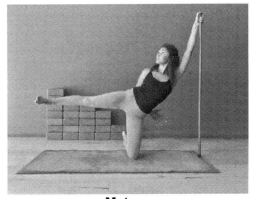

Meteor

5 deep breaths on each side

Tip: Wrap open arm behind back. Long body and leg out. Horizontal alignment. Take up space.

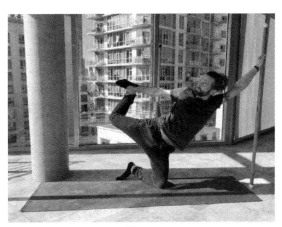

Zeus

5 - 10 deep breaths on each side

Tip: Stick and knee alignment. Strong stick hand, tummy and bottom hip. Look over top shoulder.

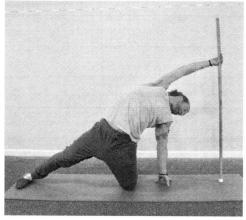

Gate

30 seconds each side

Tip: Stick, hand, knee and foot aligned on mat. Distribute body weight evenly throughout.

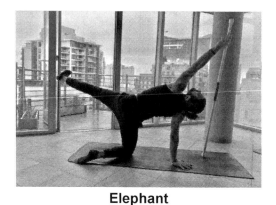

Elephant

30 seconds each side

Tip: Fun pose! Use Yogistick to create lightness throughout body. Reach and spread out.

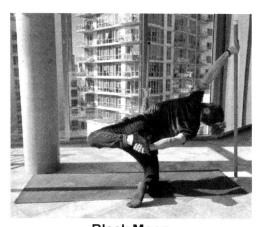

Black Moon

5 - 10 deep breaths on each side

Tip: Balance weight through core strength. Tough pose. Super focus is needed.

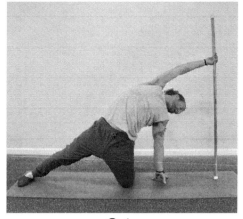

Gate
30 seconds each side
Tip: Stick, hand, knee and foot aligned on mat. Distribute body weight evenly throughout.

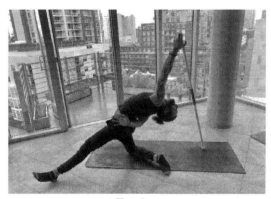

Evolve
5 - 10 deep breaths on each side
Tip: Equal weight throughout. Use top hand and extended leg to lighten body.

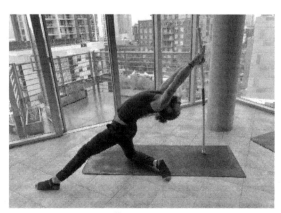

Dreamer
5 - 10 deep breaths on each side
Tip: Similar to Evolve. But with more free spirit. Space and trust.

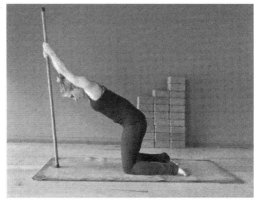

Miracle II

30 - 45 seconds with each hand on top

Tip: Squeeze imaginary block between legs. Relax head and shoulders. Hands up on stick

.

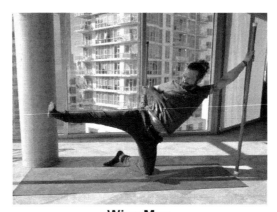

Wise Man

5 deep breaths on each side

Tip: Stack hips and grounded knee. Stick and knee alignment. Spread arm, body and leg out.

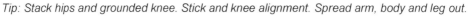

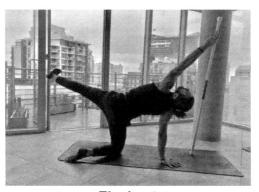

Elephant

30 seconds each side

Tip: Fun pose! Use Yogistick to create lightness throughout body. Reach and spread out.

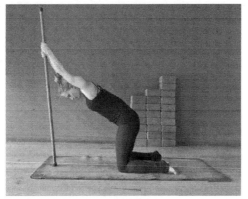

Miracle II

30 – 45 seconds with each hand on top

Tip: Squeeze imaginary block between legs. Relax head and shoulders. Hands up on stick.

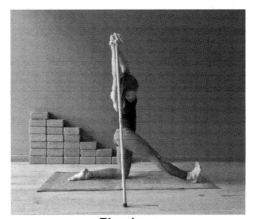

Flamingo

5 – 10 deep breaths on each side

Tip: Balance and alignment. Confidence and surrender are needed. Deep stretch.

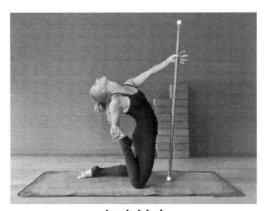

Ladybird

5 – 10 deep breaths on each side

Tip: Fun and challenging. Be easy on the low back. Less is more.

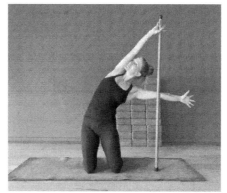

Seahorse

5 - 10 deep breaths on each side

Tip: Both knees and stick aligned on floor. Extend arms up and out. Dynamic hands.

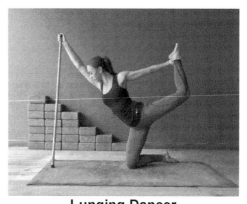

Lunging Dancer

5 - 10 deep breaths on each side

Tip: Use and focus your eyes. Find symmetry moving forward. Strong core. Not easy.

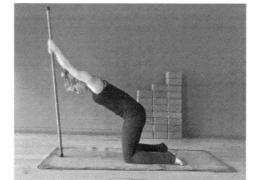

Miracle II

5 - 10 deep breaths on each side

Tip: Squeeze imaginary block between legs. Relax head and shoulders. Hands up on stick.

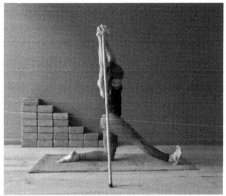

Flamingo

5 - 10 deep breaths on each side

Tip: Balance and alignment. Confidence and surrender are needed. Deep stretch.

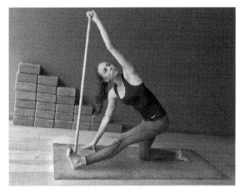

Tongue & Cheek

5 - 10 deep breaths on each side

Tip: Transition from half splits and release hand to the floor. Twist and straighten.

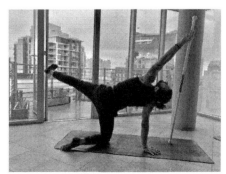

Elephant

5 - 10 deep breaths on each side

Tip: Fun pose! Use Yogistick to create lightness throughout body. Reach and spread out.

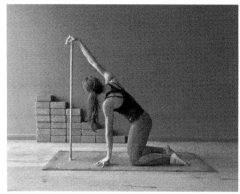

Toothpick

5 - 10 deep breaths on each side

Tip: Keep close to the stick and pancake the top hand. If possible, hips stay straight and twist up.

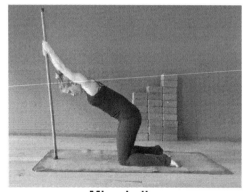

Miracle II

5 - 10 deep breaths on each side

Tip: Squeeze imaginary block between legs. Relax head and shoulders. Hands up on stick.

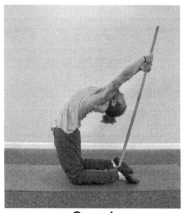

Camel

5 - 10 deep breaths on each side

Tip: Start easy. Create space for your head. Heart over knees. Hands way up. Less is more.

Triangle

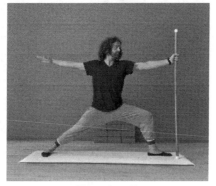

Warrior II
10 breaths on each side

Tip: Foot, stick and back heel alignment. Strong toes. Roll thighs in and up. Hands up with back hand awareness.

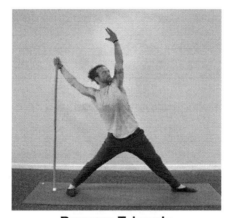

Reverse Triangle
10 breaths on each side

Tip: Be long, tall and create space. Parallel waist line to floor. Back hand up on stick. Strength from ground up.

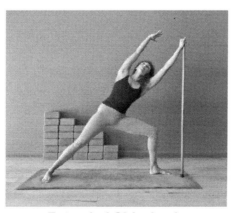

Extended Side Angle
10 breaths on each side

Tip: Think of your body as a sliding glass door. Stay in the frame and expand everywhere.

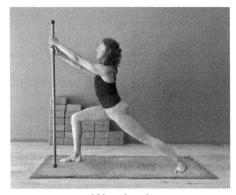

Warrior I

10 breaths on each side

Tip: Hips, chest and body aligned with stick. Grip your toes. Feel buoyant and balanced.

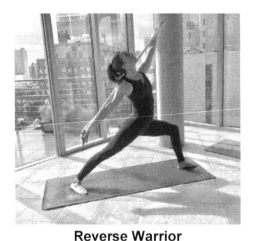

Reverse Warrior

5 - 10 breaths on each side

Tip: Build from ground up. Strength everywhere and stay balanced in both feet.

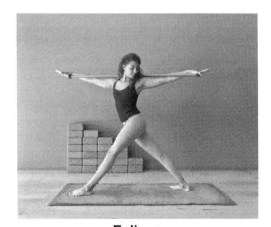

Eclipse

10 breaths on each side

Tip: Be flexible, light and strong. Twist from the core and wingspan your arms.

Triangle 2

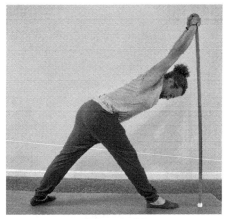

Miracle V

45 - 60 seconds on each side

Tip: Heel and stick alignment. Hips, heart and stick alignment. Strong tummy. Long arms and relax your head.

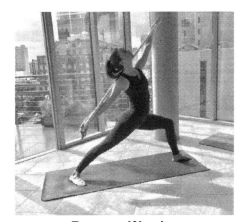

Reverse Warrior

5 -10 breaths on each side

Tip: Build from ground up. Strength everywhere and stay balanced in both feet.

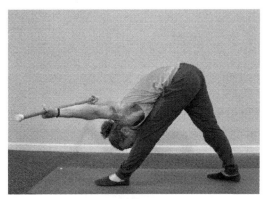

Wavelength

45 seconds on each side

Tip: Start with reverse grip and rotate over head. Tailbone and heel alignment. Lengthen spine.

Triangle 3

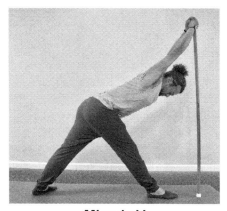

Miracle V

45 - 60 seconds on each side

Tip: Heel and stick alignment. Hips, heart and stick alignment. Strong tummy. Long arms and relax your head.

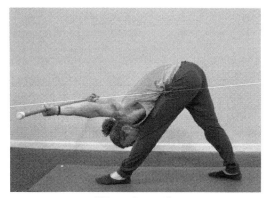

Wavelength

45 seconds on each side

Tip: Start with reverse grip and rotate over head. Tailbone and heel alignment. Lengthen spine.

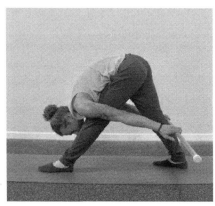

Pyramid

5 -10 breaths on each side

Tip: Start with reverse grip and extend stick down leg. Tailbone and heel alignment. Lengthen spine.

Triangle 4

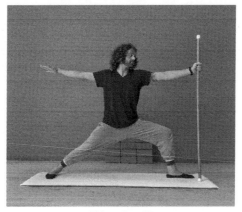

Warrior II

5 -10 breaths on each side

Tip: Foot, stick and back heel alignment. Strong toes. Roll thighs in and up. Hands up with back hand awareness.

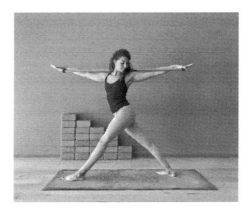

Eclipse

5 -10 breaths on each side

Tip: Be flexible, light and strong. Twist from the core and wingspan your arms.

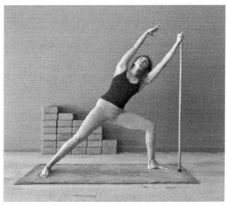

Extended Side Angle

10 breaths on each side

Tip: Think of your body as a sliding glass door. Stay in the frame and expand everywhere.

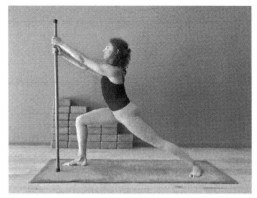

Warrior I

5 -10 breaths on each side

Tip: Hips, chest and body aligned with stick. Grip your toes. Feel buoyant and balanced.

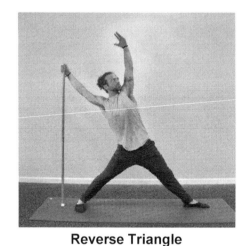

Reverse Triangle

5 -10 breaths on each side

Tip: Be long, tall and create space. Parallel waist line to floor. Back hand up on stick. Strength from ground up.

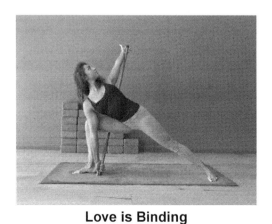

Love is Binding

5 -10 breaths on each side

Tip: See extended side angle. Start with stick near back hip and feed under body to front hand.

Belly

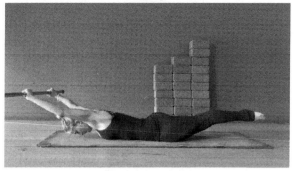

Magnetic Field

2 times, 5 -10 breaths

Tip: Press stick forward and pull feet back. Energize the entire body. Hover as much body off of the floor as possible.

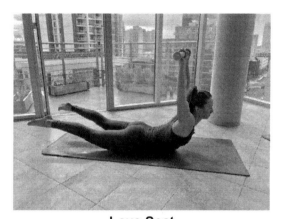

Love Seat

2 times, 5 -10 breaths

Tip: Backside core strength needed. Forward grip. Stick aligned over shoulders. Strong legs.

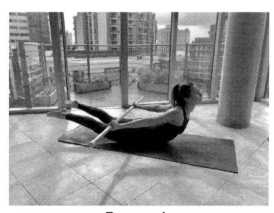

Barracuda

5-10 breaths

Tip: Let the Yogisstick pull chest forward. Scale and balance energy throughout.

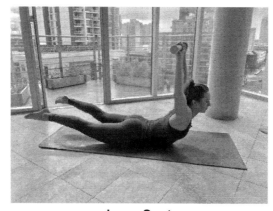

Love Seat

2 times, 5 -10 breaths

Tip: Backside core strength needed. Forward grip. Stick aligned over shoulders. Strong legs.

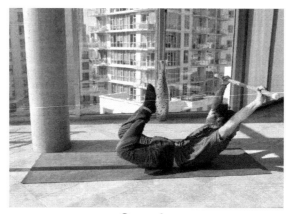

Scorpio

5 -10 breaths

Tip: Fun pose here. Bring big toes to touch and lift arms way up. Strong butt.

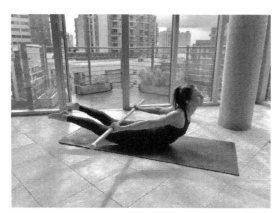

Barracuda

5-10 breaths

Tip: Let the Yogisstick pull chest forward. Scale and balance energy throughout.

Belly 2

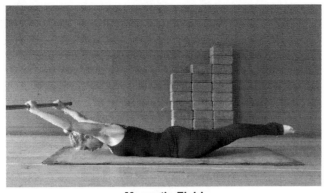

Magnetic Field
2 times, 5 -10 breaths
Tip: Press stick forward and pull feet back. Energize the entire body. Hover as much body off of the floor as possible.

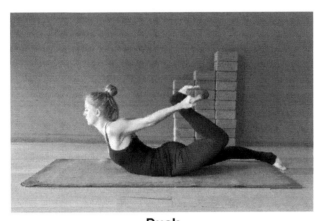

Duck
5 -10 breaths each side
Tip: Both legs are active. Lengthen and press base leg into the floor. Strong back. Pelvis down. Breathe.

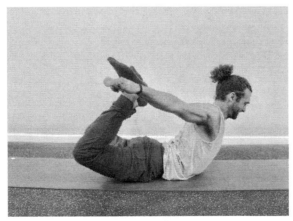

Open Heart
2 times, 5 -10 breaths
Tip: See Duck. Be warmed up. Breath often for success here and be patient.

Standing

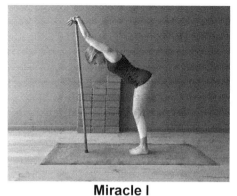

Miracle I

1 minute each hand on top

Tip: Long arms and legs. Relax head, neck and shoulders. Flex your stomach. Heavy tail bone.

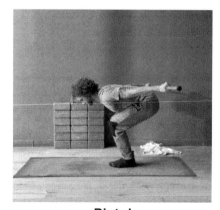

Pistol

5 - 10 deep breaths

Tip: Reverse grip. Belly to thighs. Strong legs. Long spine through your head. Press stick past tail bone

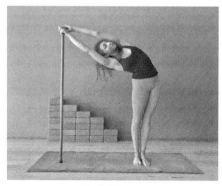

Full Moon

5 - 10 deep breaths on each side

Tip: Be sure stick and hands are at proper height. Body aligned with stick. Strong toes, legs and core.

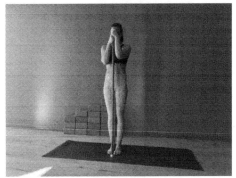

Namaste

5 - 10 deep breaths each hand on top

Tip: Close eyes, breathe well and build from the ground up. Clear your mind and become present.

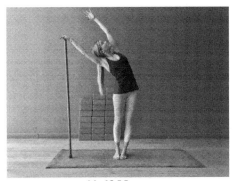

Half Moon

5 - 10 deep breaths on each side

Tip: Long body and stick alignment. Energize legs, pelvis and tummy. Stick hand way up and reach.

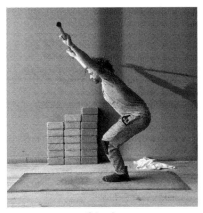

Chair

5 - 10 deep breaths

Tip: Use stick to keep arms up. Use your toes. Heavy tailbone and flex stomach. Bend knees for strong legs.

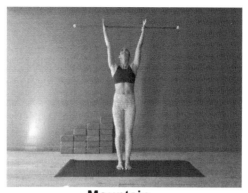

Mountain

5 - 10 deep breaths

Tip: Reach for the stars but keep your feet on the ground.

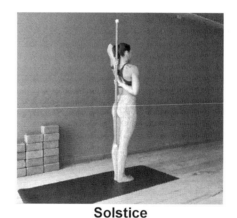

Solstice

10 deep breaths on each side

Tip: Use Yogistick to crawl hands toward each other. Grab the stick. Don't clasp fingers. Elbows inward toward body.

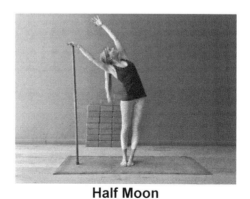

Half Moon

5 - 10 deep breaths on each side

Tip: Long body and stick alignment. Energize legs, pelvis and tummy. Stick hand way up and reach.

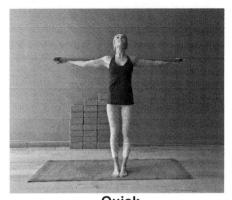

Quick

5 - 10 deep breaths

Tip: Extend arms way out and challenge expansion.

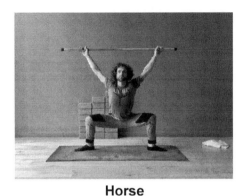

Horse

5 - 10 deep breaths

Tip: Toe, knee, heel, shoulder and stick alignment. Press stick way up. Strong body and feel buoyant.

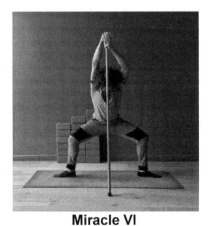

Miracle VI

10 deep breaths with each hand on top

Tip: Leg and shoulder alignment. Pelvis inward and up. Use stick to alleviate stress in feet. Pancake grip.

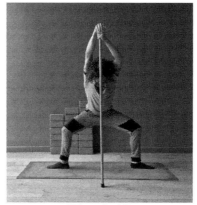

Miracle VI

10 deep breaths with each hand on top

Tip: Leg and shoulder alignment. Pelvis inward and up. Use stick to alleviate stress in feet. Pancake grip.

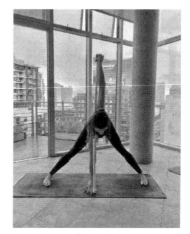

Gemini

5 - 10 deep breaths on each side

Tip: Pivot stick for alignment. Twist from stomach and try to keep hips square. Strong feet and long wingspan.

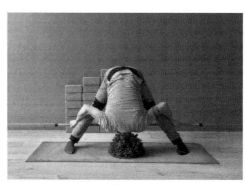

Juno

5 - 10 deep breaths

Tip: Use stick for leverage to fold deeper and use biceps. Allow blood to flow down to head.

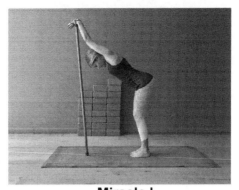

Miracle I

1 minute with each hand on top

Tip: Long arms and legs. Relax head, neck and shoulders. Flex your stomach. Heavy tail bone.

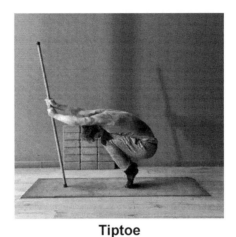

Tiptoe

5 - 10 deep breaths with each hand on top

Tip: Use stick to alleviate stress from toes. Belly to thighs. Chin over knees. Fun pose.

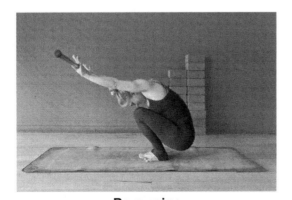

Porcupine

5 - 10 deep breaths

Tip: Harder than you think. Find comfort in uncomfort. Chin to knees. Arms higher than head and hips down.

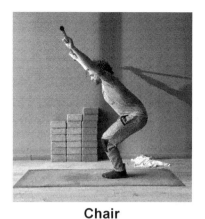

Chair

5 - 10 deep breaths

Tip: Use stick to keep arms up. Use your toes. Heavy tailbone and flex stomach. Bend knees for strong legs.

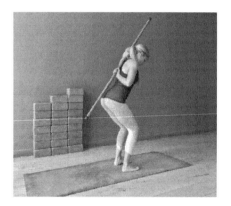

Ostrich

5 - 10 deep breaths on each side

Tip: Ankle, knee, hip and shoulder alignment. Align stick with spine and crawl hands inward.

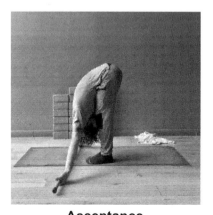

Acceptance

10 deep breaths

Tip: Reverse grip. Push chin into knees to straighten legs. Use stick leverage to release shoulders.

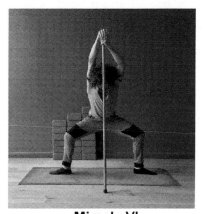

Miracle VI

10 deep breaths with each hand on top

Tip: Leg and shoulder alignment. Pelvis inward and up. Use stick to alleviate stress in feet. Pancake grip.

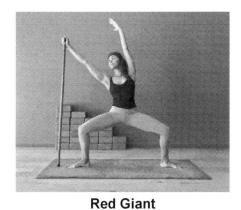

Red Giant

5 - 10 deep breaths on each side

Tip: Feet, knee and stick alignment. Keep waistline parallel to floor. Strong legs.

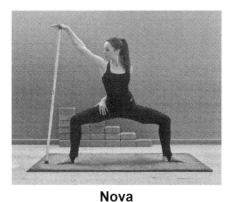

Nova

5 - 10 deep breaths on each side

Tip: Feet, knee and stick alignment. Keep waistline parallel to floor. Strong legs.

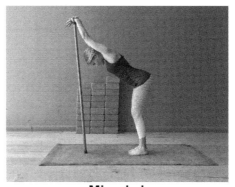

Miracle I

1 minute with each hand on top

Tip: Long arms and legs. Relax head, neck and shoulders. Flex your stomach. Heavy tail bone.

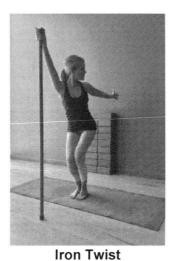

Iron Twist

5 - 10 deep breaths on each side

Tip: Strong toes and thighs. Hips forward. Use stick to pivot and twist open.

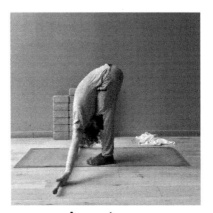

Acceptance

10 deep breaths

Tip: Reverse grip. Push chin into knees to straighten legs. Use stick leverage to release shoulders.

Standing 9

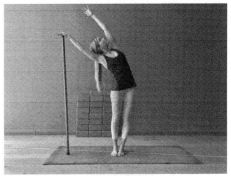

Half Moon

5 - 10 deep breaths on each side

Tip: Long body and stick alignment. Energize legs, pelvis and tummy. Stick hand way up and reach.

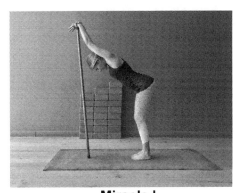

Miracle I

1 minute with each hand on top

Tip: Long arms and legs. Relax head, neck and shoulders. Flex your stomach. Heavy tail bone.

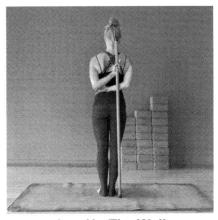

Arm Up The Wall

10 deep breaths on each side

Tip: Pivot stick near hip and heel. Fingers to elbows. Grab stick and crawl hand way up.

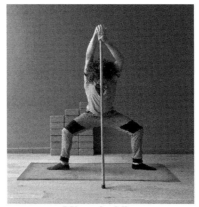

Miracle VI

10 deep breaths with each hand on top

Tip: Leg and shoulder alignment. Pelvis inward and up. Use stick to alleviate stress in feet. Pancake grip.

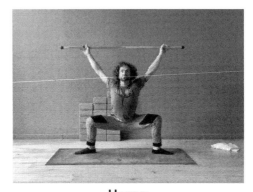

Horse

5 - 10 deep breaths

Tip: Toe, knee, heel, shoulder and stick alignment. Press stick way up. Strong body and feel buoyant.

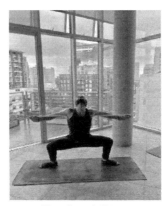

Evolved Star

5 - 10 deep breaths

Tip: Be warmed up. Impala arms with horse body. Strong core and legs are a must.

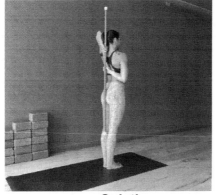

Solstice

10 deep breaths on each side

Tip: Use Yogistick to crawl hands toward each other. Grab the stick. Don't clasp fingers. Elbows inward toward body.

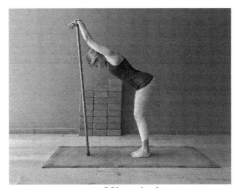

Miracle I

1 minute with each hand on top

Tip: Long arms and legs. Relax head, neck and shoulders. Flex your stomach. Heavy tail bone.

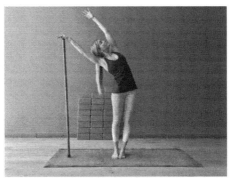

Half Moon

10 deep breaths on each side

Tip: Long body and stick alignment. Energize legs, pelvis and tummy. Stick hand way up and reach.

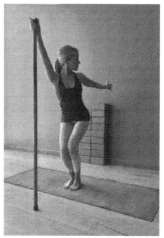

Iron Twist

5 - 10 deep breaths on each side

Tip: Strong toes and thighs. Hips forward. Align stick with belly button. Pivot stick and twist open.

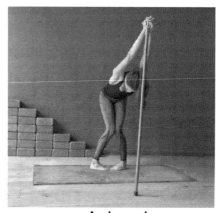

Awkward

15 – 20 deep breaths on each side

Tip: Big toes touch. Seal thighs from your belly button to your knees. Coil belly and relax head.

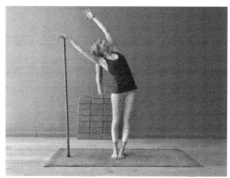

Half Moon

5 - 10 deep breaths on each side

Tip: Long body and stick alignment. Energize legs, pelvis and tummy. Stick hand way up and reach.

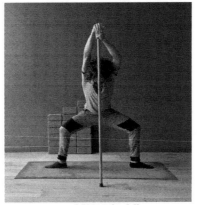

Miracle VI

10 deep breaths with each hand on top

Tip: Leg and shoulder alignment. Pelvis inward and up. Use stick to alleviate stress in feet. Pancake grip.

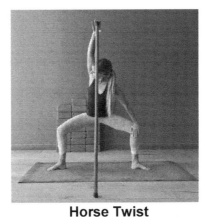

Horse Twist

5 - 10 deep breaths on each side

Tip: Horse legs. Scoop pelvis inward and up. Use stick to pivot and twist.

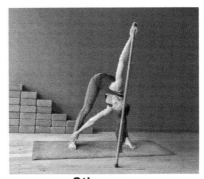

Stingray

5 - 10 deep breaths on each side

Tip: Use your legs and square hips. Use stick to pivot. Catch ankle and twist.

Lunge

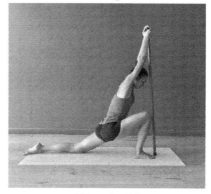

Miracle IV

30 - 45 seconds on each side

Tip: Great stretch. Meridian of body and stick alignment. Energize and square hips. Hands way up.

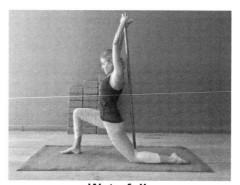

Waterfall

5 - 10 deep breaths on each side

Tip: Align stick with spine and parachute your hands. Bend front leg and press hips forward.

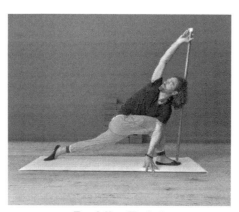

Buddha Twist

5 - 10 deep breaths on each side

Tip: Meridian of body and stick alignment. Untuck back toe and energize hips. Fun pose.

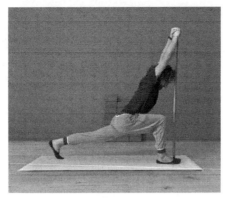

Goat

5 - 10 deep breaths on each side

Tip: Meridian of body and stick alignment. Challenge vertical space. Canopy hands. Relax head.

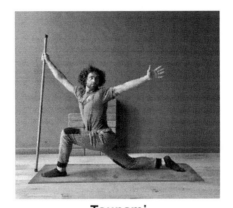

Tsunami

5 - 10 deep breaths on each side

Tip: Meridian of body and stick alignment. Peg stick down and twist with core.

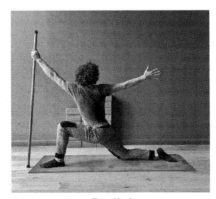

Radial

5 - 10 deep breaths on each side

Tip: Meridian of body and stick alignment. Peg stick down and twist with core.

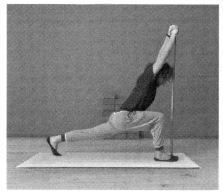

Goat

5 - 10 deep breaths on each side

Tip: Meridian of body and stick alignment. Challenge vertical space. Canopy hands. Relax head.

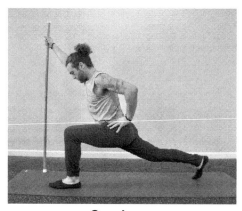

Capricorn

5 - 10 deep breaths on each side

Tip: Use Yogistick to lighten feet. Take up lots of space above your mat. Pivot stick up and out.

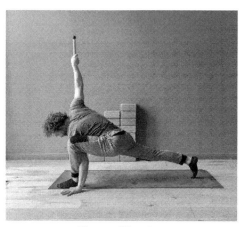

Open Cluster

5 - 10 deep breaths on each side

Tip: Use stick as leverage to wrap under and outside of foot. Hips are parallel to your mat.

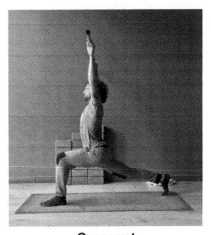

Crescent

5 deep breaths on each side

Tip: Feet hip width apart in lunge. Hip, shoulder and stick alignment. Strong tummy.

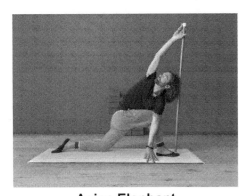

Asian Elephant

5 - 10 deep breaths on each side

Tip: Meridian of body and stick alignment. Elbow over thigh. Pelvis forward and top hand way up.

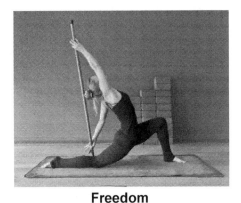

Freedom

5 - 10 deep breaths on each side

Tip: Meridian of body and stick alignment. Use stick to create lightness. Top hand way up.

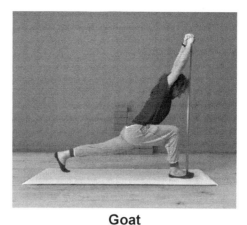

Goat

5 - 10 deep breaths on each side

Tip: Meridian of body and stick alignment. Challenge vertical space. Canopy hands. Relax head.

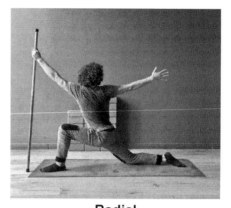

Radial

5 - 10 deep breaths on each side

Tip: Meridian of body and stick alignment. Peg stick down and twist with core.

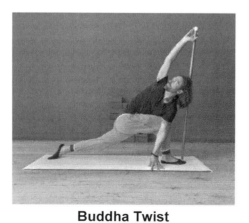

Buddha Twist

5 - 10 deep breaths on each side

Tip: Great stretch. Meridian of body and stick alignment. Energize and square hips. Hands way up.

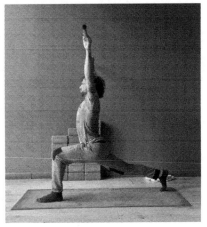

Crescent

5 - deep breaths on each side

Tip: Feet hip width apart in lunge. Hip, shoulder and stick alignment. Strong tummy.

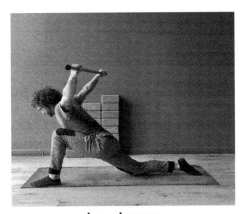

Low Lunge

5 - 10 deep breaths on each side

Tip: Lots of space. Reverse grip. Include shoulder rotations with Yogistick.

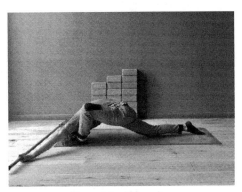

Humble Warrior

5 - 10 deep breaths on each side

Tip: From low lunge, nudge inside shoulder inside inner thigh. Square shoulders forward.

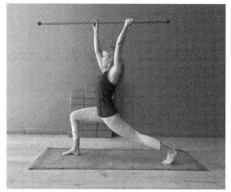

Xena Warrior
5 - 10 deep breaths on each side switching grips
Tip: Wide stance with meridian of body and stick alignment. Feel buoyant and press stick up with hands.

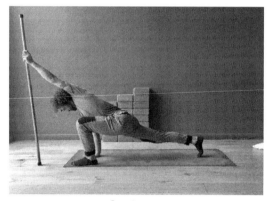

Sprinter
10 deep breaths on each side
Tip: Longest line available from back heel to top hand. Equal energy through hands and feet.

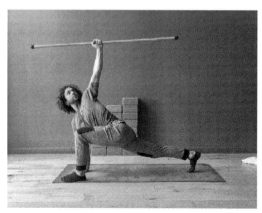

Javelin
5 - 10 deep breaths on each side
Tip: Press stick upward. Twist from balanced hands and feet.

Lunge 7

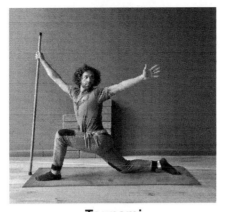

Tsunami

5 - 10 deep breaths on each side

Tip: Meridian of body and stick alignment. Peg stick down and twist with core.

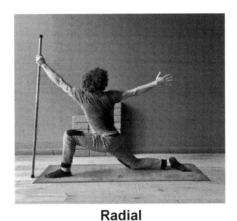

Radial

5 - 10 deep breaths on each side

Tip: Meridian of body and stick alignment. Peg stick down and twist with core.

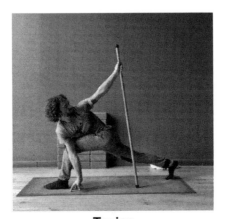

Trojan

10 deep breaths on each side

Tip: Use stick to create space with arm twisting over thigh. Look over top shoulder.

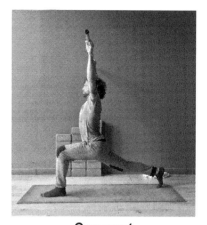

Crescent

5 deep breaths on each side

Tip: Feet hip width apart in lunge. Hip, shoulder and stick alignment. Strong tummy.

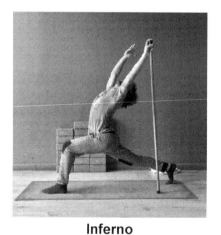

Inferno

5 deep breaths on each side

Tip: Be warmed up. Stick aligned with hip and bent leg. Heart over pelvis. Think up and out.

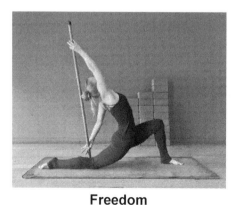

Freedom

5 - 10 deep breaths on each side

Tip: Meridian of body and stick alignment. Use stick to create lightness. Top hand way up.

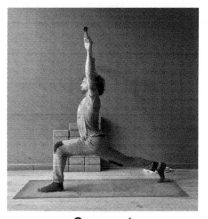

Crescent

5 deep breaths on each side

Tip: Feet hip width apart in lunge. Hip, shoulder and stick alignment. Strong tummy.

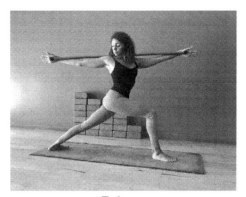

Falcon

5 - 10 deep breaths on each side

Tip: Fun pose. Knob hands over end tips. Twist from spine and core strength. Strong legs.

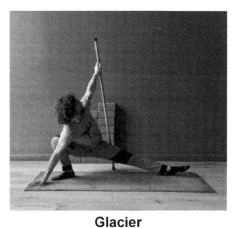

Glacier

5 deep breaths on each side

Tip: Space arms out with YogiStick. Be agile. Twist upward with hips and core.

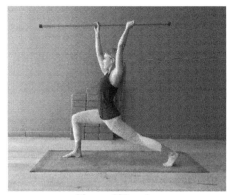

Xena Warrior

5 - 10 deep breaths on each side switching grips

Tip: Wide stance with meridian of body and stick alignment. Feel buoyant and press stick up with hands.

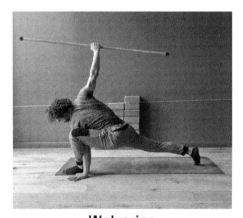

Wolverine

5 - 10 deep breaths on each side

Tip: Strong spacious legs. Heart and chest down. Use stick as a weight and press up.

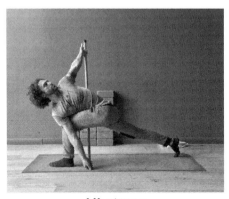

Albatross

5 - 10 deep breaths on each side

Tip: Best to start from a knee. Thread stick under body toward bottom hand. Use stick alignment

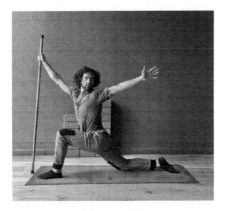

Tsunami

5 - 10 deep breaths on each side
Tip: Meridian of body and stick alignment. Peg stick down and twist with core.

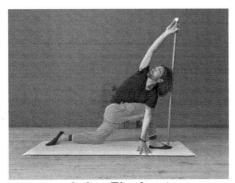

Asian Elephant

5 - 10 deep breaths on each side
Tip: Meridian of body and stick alignment. Elbow over thigh. Pelvis forward and top hand way up.

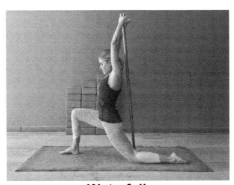

Waterfall

5 - 10 deep breaths on each side
Tip: Align stick with spine and parachute your hands. Bend front leg and press hips forward.

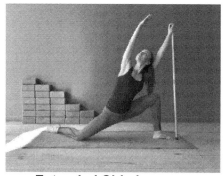

Extended Side Lunge
10 deep breaths on each side
Tip: Think of your body as a sliding glass door. Stay in the frame and expand everywhere.

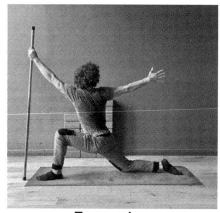

Tsunami
5 - 10 deep breaths on each side
Tip: Meridian of body and stick alignment. Peg stick down and twist with core.

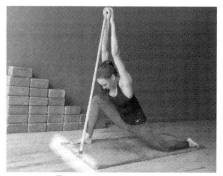

Runners Lunge
5 - 10 deep breaths on each side
Tip: Wide stance. Lots of width space between front heel and back knee. Hands up and relax head.

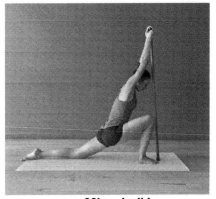

Miracle IV

30 - 45 seconds on each side

Tip: Great stretch. Meridian of body and stick alignment. Energize and square hips. Hands way up.

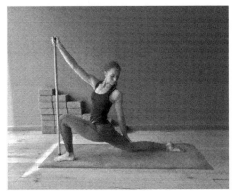

Exalted Warrior

5 - 10 deep breaths on each side

Tip: Be warmed up. Belly button forward and use your legs. Use stick to twist, wrap hand and lighten backbend.

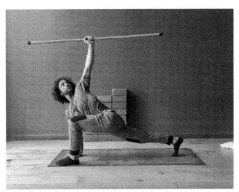

Javelin

5 - 10 deep breaths on each side

Tip: Wingspan arms. Twist from balanced hands and feet.

Balancing

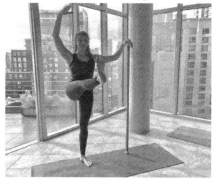

Ballerina

5 - 10 breaths on each side

Tip: Use stick to stand upright. Hip and stick alignment. Take up space with lifting arm and leg.

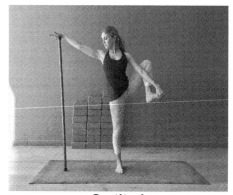

Gratitude

5 - 10 breaths on each side

Tip: Have fun. Stand tall and confident balancing with the Yogistick. Patience for progression.

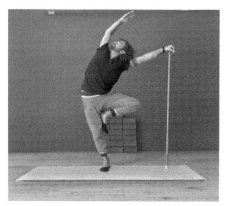

Tree

30 seconds on each side

Tip: Have fun. Use stick to place soul of foot in upper inner thigh. Both arms up and out.

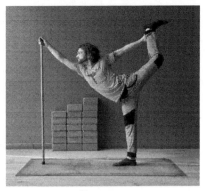

Dancer

30 - 45 seconds on each side

Tip: Fun pose. Use stick to carry heart forward but remaining grounded. Kick shin up and back.

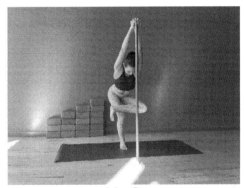

Humble Gypsy

1 minute each side

Tip: Pivot stick in line with your hips and close to your body. Bend standing leg. Open your hips. Hands way up.

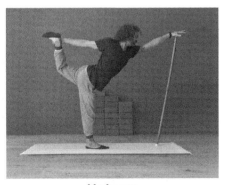

Unicorn

30 - 45 seconds on each side

Tip: Pancake grip. Opposite hand catching opposite foot. Chest and pelvis forward.

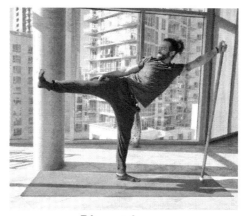

Dhurva Lama

30 - 45 seconds on each side

Tip: Grounded foot and stick alignment. Look down side of body. Improve balance here.

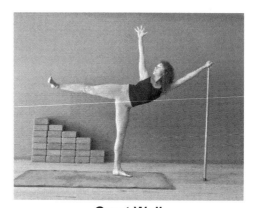

Great Wall

30 - 45 seconds on each side

Tip: So much fun. Align entire body along with stick. Roll top leg up and out. Look towards back leg. Lots of space.

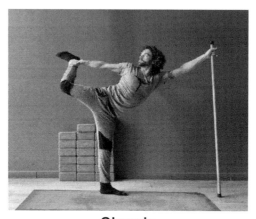

Olympic

5 - 10 breaths on each side

Tip: See Dancer pose. Catch outer ankle. Twist body up and away from floor.

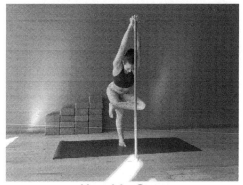

Humble Gypsy

1 minute each side

Tip: Pivot stick in line with your hips and close to your body. Bend standing leg. Open your hips. Hands way up.

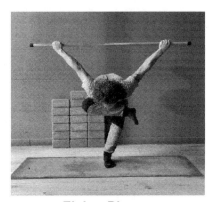

Flying Pigeon

5 - 10 breaths on each side

Tip: Reverse grip. Bend standing leg. Move chest towards shin. Long arms. Look down.

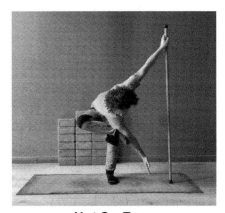

Not So Easy

5 breaths on each side

Tip: Feet, shoulder and stick alignment. Use stick for leveraging tricep over arch of foot.

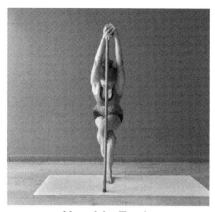

Humble Eagle

30 seconds on each side

Tip: One of my favorite poses. Use stick for balance. Double stack grip. Keep foot wrapped up.

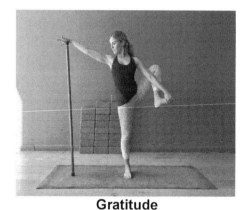

Gratitude

5 - 10 breaths on each side

Tip: Have fun. Stand tall and confident balancing with the Yogistick. Patience for progression.

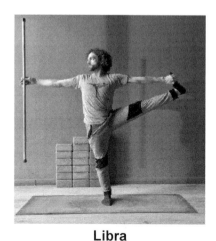

Libra

10 breaths on each side

Tip: From gratitude pose, extend foot up and away from body. Be warmed up. Look toward stick

Balancing 5

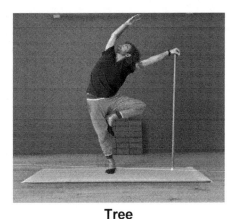

Tree

30 seconds on each side

Tip: Have fun. Use stick to place soul of foot in upper inner thigh. Both arms up and out.

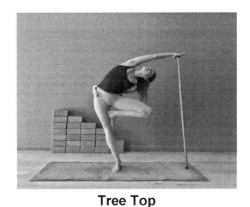

Tree Top

5 - 10 breaths on each side

Tip: Be warmed up. See tree pose and switch hands. Body and stick alignment. Pelvis forward.

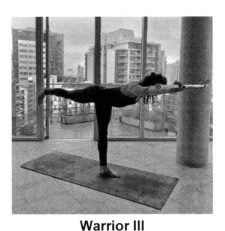

Warrior III

30 - 45 seconds with each hand on top

Tip: Mountain pose arms and press stick out. Elongate throughout meridian line. Press and pull lifted heel back.

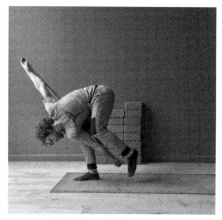

Bind and Balance

5 - 10 breaths on each side

Tip: See love is binding. Shift weight and balance on front foot. Bring stick around leg and wingspan arms along stick

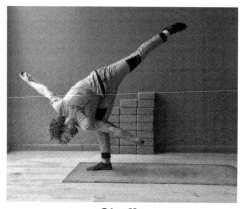

Giraffe

5 breaths on each side

Tip: Stare at standing big toe. Extend back leg up and away from bind and balance pose.

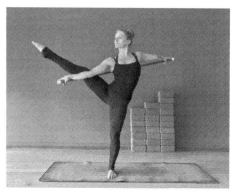

Birds of Paradise

5 - 10 breaths on each side

Tip: Use stick bind to keep leg elevated. Grow from the ground up. Stand tall. Hips forward.

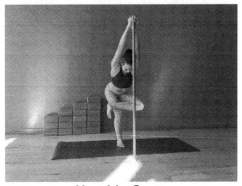

Humble Gypsy

1 minute each side

Tip: Pivot stick in line with your hips and close to your body. Bend standing leg. Open your hips. Hands way up.

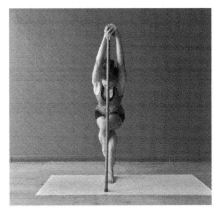

Humble Eagle

30 seconds on each side

Tip: One of my favorite poses. Use stick for balance. Double stack grip. Keep foot wrapped up.

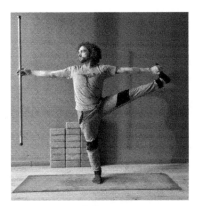

Libra

10 breaths on each side

Tip: From gratitude pose, extend foot up and away from body. Be warmed up. Look toward stick

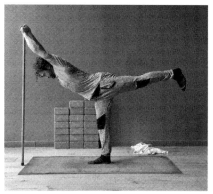

Balancing Stick

30 - 45 seconds with each hand on top

Tip: Signature Pose. Elongate throughout meridian line. Press and pull lifted heel back.

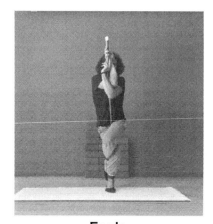

Eagle

30 seconds on each side

Tip: Wrap arms around stick first, then your legs. Fun challenging pose. See humble gypsy pose.

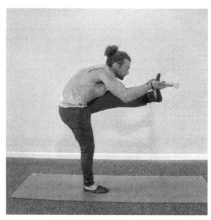

SSLFK

5 - 10 breaths on each side

Tip: Light hands and energy using stick. Use core to lift leg and extend outward. Breathe.

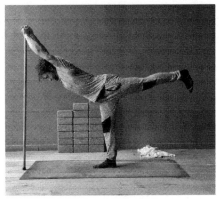

Balancing Stick

30 - 45 seconds with each hand on top

Tip: Signature Pose. Elongate throughout meridian line. Press and pull lifted heel back.

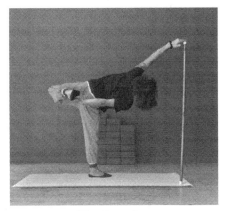

Challenging

5 - 10 deep breaths on each side

Tip: Tough pose. Standing leg, top arm and stick alignment. Lots of trust. Bottom hand catch arch of foot.

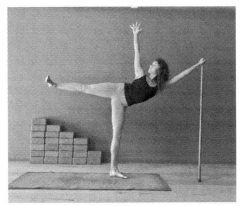

Great Wall

5 - 10 deep breaths on each side

Tip: So much fun. Align entire body along with stick. Roll top leg up and out. Look towards back leg. Lots of space.

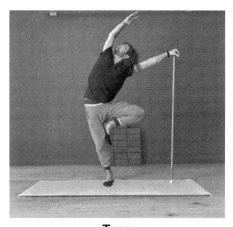

Tree

30 seconds on each side

Tip: Have fun. Use stick to place soul of foot in upper inner thigh. Both arms up and out.

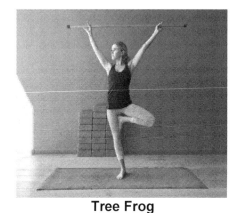

Tree Frog

30 seconds on each side

Tip: From tree pose, extend stick over head and press up. Stick, head, shoulder and hip aligned

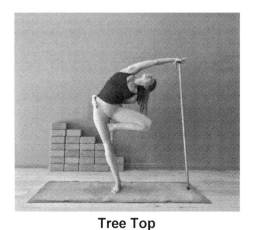

Tree Top

30 seconds on each side

Tip: Be warmed up. See tree pose and switch hands. Body and stick alignment. Pelvis forward.

Balancing 11

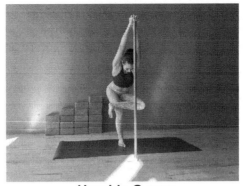

Humble Gypsy

1 minute each side

Tip: Pivot stick in line with your hips and close to your body. Bend standing leg. Open your hips. Hands way up.

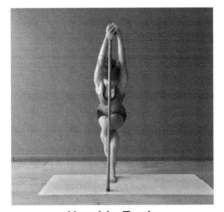

Humble Eagle

30 seconds on each side

Tip: One of my favorite poses. Use stick for balance. Double stack grip. Keep foot wrapped up.

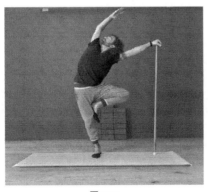

Tree

30 seconds on each side

Tip: Have fun. Use stick to place soul of foot in upper inner thigh. Both arms up and out.

Arm Balance

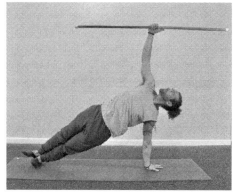

Side Plank

5 - 10 breaths on each side

Tip: Bottom hand and foot alignment. Bump top hip way up. Keep stick aligned with body.

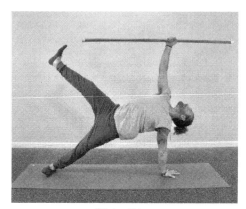

Side Star

5 - 10 breaths on each side

Tip: From side plank, slightly bend top leg and lift with strength and comfort. Body & stick align.

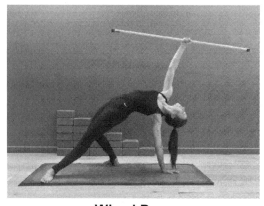

Wheel Prep

5 - 10 breaths on each side

Tip: From either of these planks, place top foot back and down outside of mat. Lift pelvis up.

Arm Balance 1

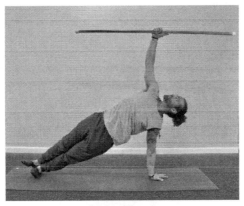

Side Plank

5 - 10 breaths on each side

Tip: Bottom hand and foot alignment. Bump top hip way up. Keep stick aligned with body.

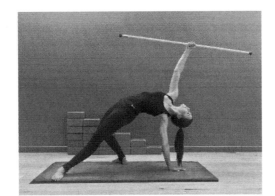

Wheel Prep

5 - 10 breaths on each side

Tip: From side plank, place top foot back and down outside of mat. Lift pelvis upward.

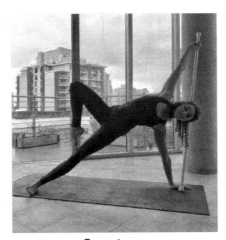

Spectrum

5 - 10 breaths on each side

Tip: From wheel prep, pivot stick down near balancing hand. Slide foot to inner thigh. Be light.

Mixed

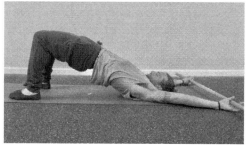

Bridge

3 times, 5 - 10 deep breaths

Tip: Grab the floor with your feet. Toes, knees, hips, shoulders aligned. Strong core and pelvis.

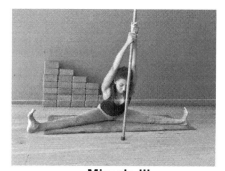

Miracle III

I minute with each hand on top

Tip: Hands up and pivot top of stick away from you. Strong hands and tummy. Relax your head and toes.

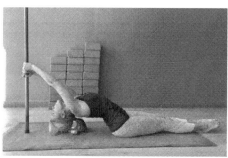

Fish

30 - 45 seconds with each hand on top

Tip: Less is more here. Create space to release your head back between your arms.

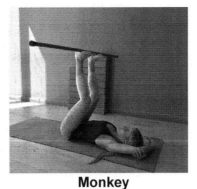

Monkey
Hold for 1 minute and switch grip
Tip: Tailbone slightly off the floor. Bend your knees and practice patience.

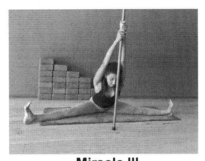

Miracle III
I minute with each hand on top
Tip: Hands up and pivot top of stick away from you. Strong hands and tummy. Relax your head and toes.

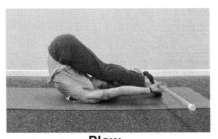

Plow
3 times, 5 deep breaths
Tip: Breathing here is everything. Stay longer and reap the benefits.

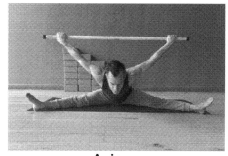

Axis

30 - 45 seconds

Tip: Strong stomach. Hing from hips like a door. Reverse grip. Press arms up, back and overhead.

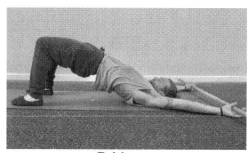

Bridge

3 times, 5 - 10 deep breaths

Tip: Grab the floor with your feet. Toes, knees, hips, shoulders aligned. Strong core and pelvis.

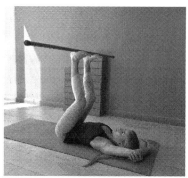

Monkey

Hold for 1 minute and switch grip

Tip: Tailbone slightly off the floor. Bend your knees and practice patience.

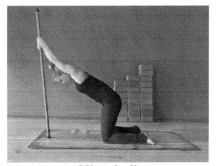

Miracle II

30 - 45 seconds with each hand on top

Tip: Squeeze imaginary block between legs. Relax head and shoulders. Hands up on stick.

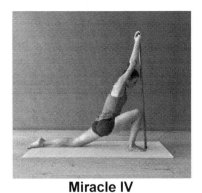

Miracle IV

30 - 45 seconds on each side

Tip: Great stretch. Meridian of body and stick alignment. Energize and square hips. Hands way up.

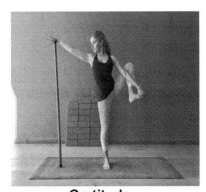

Gratitude

5 - 10 breaths on each side

Tip: Have fun. Stand tall and confident balancing with the Yogistick. Patience for progression

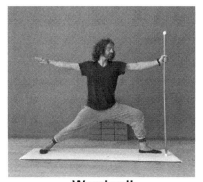

Warrior II

10 breaths on each side

Tip: Foot, stick and back heel alignment. Strong toes. Roll thighs in and up. Hands up with back hand awareness.

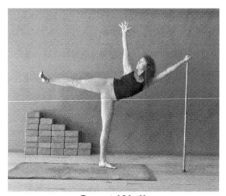

Great Wall

30 - 45 seconds on each side

Tip: So much fun. Align entire body along with stick. Roll top leg up and out. Look towards back leg. Lots of space.

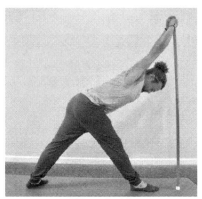

Miracle V

45 - 60 seconds on each side

Tip: Heel and stick alignment. Hips, heart and stick alignment. Strong tummy. Long arms and relax your head.

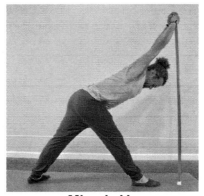

Miracle V

45 - 60 seconds on each side

Tip: Heel and stick alignment. Hips, heart and stick alignment. Strong tummy. Long arms and relax your head.

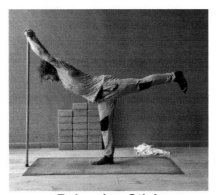

Balancing Stick

30 - 45 seconds with each hand on top

Tip: Signature Pose. Elongate throughout meridian line. Press and pull lifted heel back.

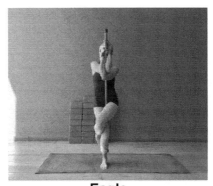

Eagle

30 seconds on each side

Tip: Wrap arms around stick first, then your legs. Fun challenging pose. See humble gypsy pose.

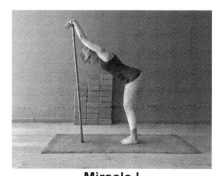

Miracle I

1 minute with each hand on top

Tip: Long arms and legs. Relax head, neck and shoulders. Flex your stomach. Heavy tail bone.

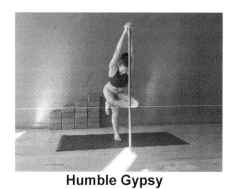

Humble Gypsy

1 minute each side

Tip: Pivot stick in line with your hips and close to your body. Bend standing leg. Open your hips. Hands way up.

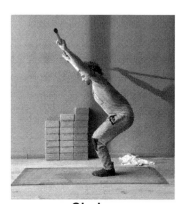

Chair

5 - 10 deep breaths

Tip: Use stick to keep arms up. Use your toes. Heavy tailbone and flex stomach. Bend knees for strong legs.

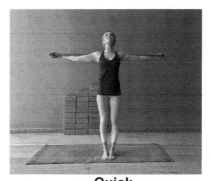

Quick

5 - 10 deep breaths

Tip: Extend arms way out and challenge expansion.

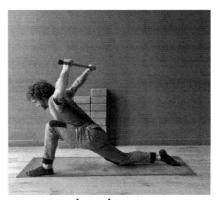

Low Lunge

5 - 10 deep breaths on each side

Tip: Lots of space. Reverse grip. Include shoulder rotations with Yogistick.

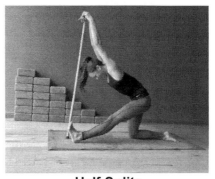

Half Splits

5 - 10 deep breaths on each side

Tip: Line up stick with nose. Long arms. Use core for balance. Keep hips in a frame.

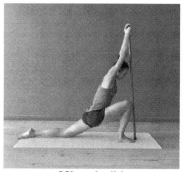

Miracle IV

30 - 45 seconds on each side

Tip: Great stretch. Meridian of body and stick alignment. Energize and square hips. Hands way up.

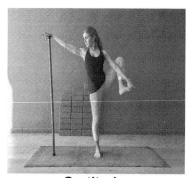

Gratitude

5 - 10 breaths on each side

Tip: Have fun. Stand tall and confident balancing with the Yogistick. Patience for progression

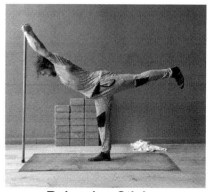

Balancing Stick

30 - 45 seconds with each hand on top

Tip: Signature Pose. Elongate throughout meridian line. Press and pull lifted heel back.

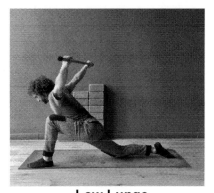

Low Lunge

5 - 10 deep breaths on each side

Tip: Lots of space. Reverse grip. Include shoulder rotations with Yogistick.

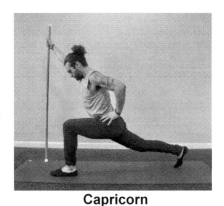

Capricorn

5 - 10 deep breaths on each side

Tip: Use Yogistick to lighten feet. Take up lots of space above your mat. Pivot stick up and out.

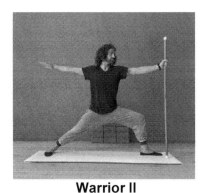

Warrior II

10 breaths on each side

Tip: Foot, stick and back heel alignment. Strong toes. Roll thighs in and up. Hands up with back hand awareness.

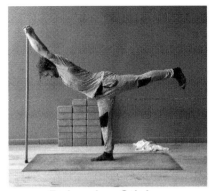

Balancing Stick

30 - 45 seconds with each hand on top

Tip: Signature Pose. Elongate throughout meridian line. Press and pull lifted heel back.

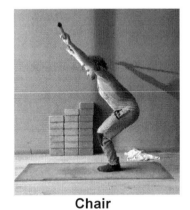

Chair

5 - 10 deep breaths

Tip: Use stick to keep arms up. Use your toes. Heavy tailbone and flex stomach. Bend knees for strong legs.

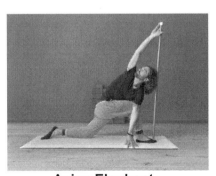

Asian Elephant

5 - 10 deep breaths on each side

Tip: Meridian of body and stick alignment. Elbow over thigh. Pelvis forward and top hand way up.

Mixed 11

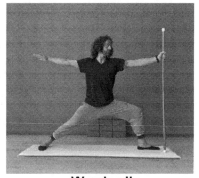

Warrior II

10 breaths on each side

Tip: Foot, stick and back heel alignment. Strong toes. Roll thighs in and up. Hands up with back hand awareness.

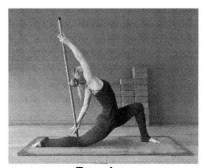

Freedom

5 - 10 deep breaths on each side

Tip: Meridian of body and stick alignment. Use stick to create lightness. Top hand way up.

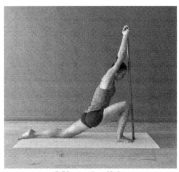

Miracle IV

30 - 45 seconds on each side

Tip: Great stretch. Meridian of body and stick alignment. Energize and square hips. Hands way up.

Yogistick Grips and Holds

Pancake

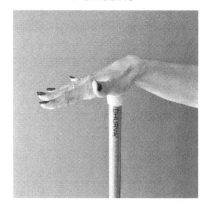

Double Stack

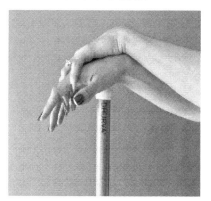

Fist Grab

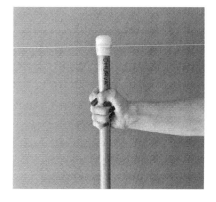

Double Fist

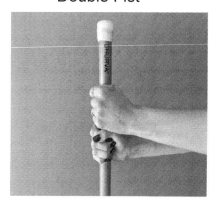

Fish Hook

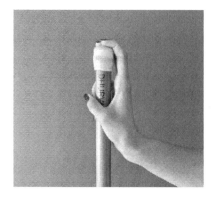

Thumb Hold

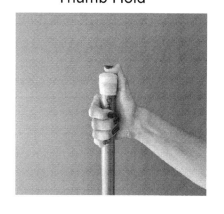

Thumb Hold

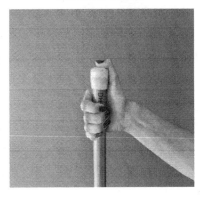

Forward Grip

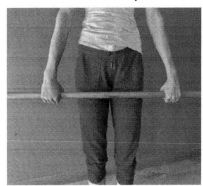

Tweezer Hold

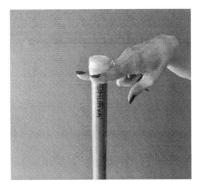

Reverse Grip

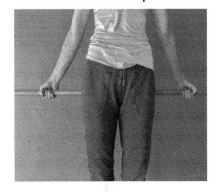

A - OK Hold

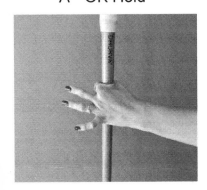

Bicep Grip

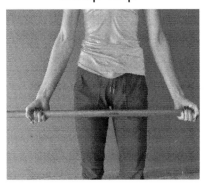

Canopy Hands

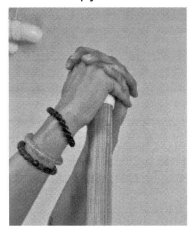

Solstice Arms

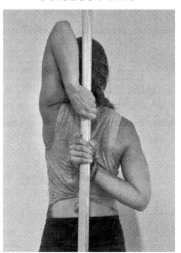

Serpent Arm

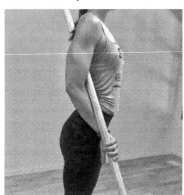

Dhurva Impressions

Physical
* Room temperature : 81-85 degrees (if studio is capable)
* Keep stick on either side of the mat (most of the time)
* Space students out. Space matters
* Drop students to a knee (low lunge) first, before going into high lunge/crescent
* Be clear on stick placement
* Be clear with hand grip on stick
* Walk the room with the stick
* Shoulders, Hips, Core every class
* Hit core hard at least 2 times in each class

Teacher
* Teach class & each pose from "the ground up" mentality
* Lead flows and movements with left side first
* Cue from the question "How can this stick help me?" Balance, strengthen, posture etc...
* Use your Miracles
* Be creative
* Refer to your books

Culture
* Enter and prep the room before any student enters prior to class "always/most of the time". Students should feel the teacher's presence in the room before they set up their mat.
* Music will flow with the flow
* Balance
* Aid, Teach, Challenge
* Black, Grey and white outfit colors

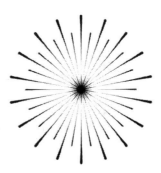

28338192R00083

Made in the USA
Columbia, SC
10 October 2018